In Search of Somatic Therapy

Setsuko Tsuchiya

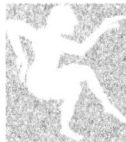

Savant Books and Publications
Honolulu, HI, USA
2017

Published in the USA by Savant Books and Publications
2630 Kapiolani Blvd #1601
Honolulu, HI 96826
http://www.savantbooksandpublications.com

Printed in the USA

Edited by David Shinsato
Cover by Daniel S. Janik

13-digit ISBN (EAN): 9780997247237

This book is primarily non-fictional; though the information conveyed comes from different sources, every effort has been made to make this work as accurate as possible. However, there may remain mistakes, both typographical and in content. Information conveyed is current up to the printing date.

Zachary M. Oliver, Randall H. James, Daniel S. Janik, Albert Franz, Roger Izumigawa and Anne Ho kindly reviewed this work.

Dedication

To Drs. Randall H. James and Daniel S. Janik, who first introduced me to the broader field of somatic therapy, and Albert Franz who introduced me to dance.

Acknowledgements

Thanks to Daniel S. Janik MD PhD, Fellow of the American College of Preventive Medicine and American Association of Integrative Medicine, my competitive DanceSport partner and champion of the neurobiological approach to learning, who inspired me to see somatic therapy in a different light and who critically reviewed this work. Also, thanks to Randall H. James DO, Diplomate in Physical Medicine and Rehabilitation, Occupational Medicine, Acupuncture and Integrative Medicine, and former President of Hawaii College of Health Sciences, who took the time to teach me the intricacies of medically-based Swedish trigger point sports massage and Reiki energy manipulation, different forms I was to learn later, of somatic therapy, and for his willingness to critically review this work. Special thanks to my colleague, Dane E. Musick LMT, who helped advance my massage skills to the point where I began questioning what the "core" elements of massage therapy, and thereby somatic therapy were.

Special thanks also to Mr. Albert Franz, Seven Times North American Ten Dance Champion, International DanceSport Adjudicator and my coach, for introducing me to the very best of keen amateur and competitive DanceSport, and thereby to dance as another form of somatic therapy. Thanks also to Mr. Geoffrey Fells, International DanceSport Adjudicator and former Organizer of the Hawaii Star Ball, in which I have had the pleasure of both competing and serving as liaison to amateur and professional Japanese DanceSport competitors. It was during my long association with Mr. Roger Izumigawa, an enthusiastic supporter of the University of Hawaii DanceSport Club and Challenge, and Hawaii Aloha State Games, that I felt compelled to look closely at the various dance syllabi and competition rules and how they related to DanceSport, dance therapy and ultimately somatic therapy.

This acknowledgement wouldn't be complete, however, without personally thanking Ms. Anne Ho, twice USA Dance National Amateur Ballroom Vice Champion and World USA Representative to the World DanceSport Federation Amateur Ballroom Senior II and III World Championships, for helping me not just apply what I'd learned from dance, but, through dance, making me experience somatic therapy firsthand. I would also like to thank Zachary M. Oliver EdD, Argosy University Institutional Vice President and my master's degree advisor, as well as Lewis Mehl-Madrona MD PhD and Barbara Mainguy MA MFA of the Coyote Institute, Orono, Maine, and Declan J. Devereaux DDS of Ala Moana Dental Care, Honolulu, Hawaii, for their advice. Finally, I would like to thank Ms. Ruth R. Janik for believing in me and supporting me throughout my long and difficult journey in search of somatic therapy.

Table of Contents

Foreward

I was delighted when Setsuko asked me to write a brief foreward to introduce her journey in search of somatic therapy. As a physician, I have always felt that there must be a definitive physical foundation underlying the continuously developing psychological "therapies." Physicians since Hippocrates began debating this under the general rubric of "the laying on of hands." Yet, despite centuries of experience and debate, the actual physical elements that make up this powerful fundamental phenomenon are still poorly understood.

I recall one night after a particularly long and difficult shift in a Newborn Intensive Care Unit, hearing the terms "piss-poor protoplasm" (referring to a patient's inability to respond to medications, or more generally, to be unable to heal him or herself) and "the touch of the black hand" (referring to the seeming absence of whatever made the laying on of hands therapeutic). I recall pondering throughout the next day the implications of these two phrases. It wasn't, however, until Setsuko asked me recently what *I* thought was the essence of "somatic" in the term "somatic therapy" (referred to these days in my profession collectively as Complementary and Alternative Medical or CAM therapies), a relatively new field she was exploring as part of a master's degree, that I remembered the profound shift in my thinking that occurred as a result of that day in the ICU twenty years prior. In short, my rather narrow "medical" appreciation of the laying on of hands once again began rapidly expanding as I reconsidered, in a more general light, what the fundamental physical elements of the many differently named somatic therapies *I* was using in my practice might be.

I found myself becoming quite excited. I think my excitement may have surprised her, making her initially wonder if sharing this question with a *physician* had been the right thing to do. Exactly how right and appropriate would be slowly revealed during the next ten years working side-by-side with her as her competition dance partner as she doggedly investigated this important question from every possible angle, from that of dance, medical massage therapy, dance movement therapy and finally from her own reconstructed definition of somatic therapy, in the process integrating the myriad different theories, types, forms, formats and approaches into a single, common one. This book you hold in your hands represents, in my opinion, a fundamental breakthrough in understanding the true foundations of somatic therapy, where the emphasis at last returns to the somatic, rather than its medical or psychological aspects. In doing so, I hope it will begin, in you, the reader, a reinvestigation into the identity, meaning and evolution of somatic therapy and its unique place in the therapeutic laying on of hands.

- Dr. Daniel S. Janik MD PhD (2016)

Chapter 1
It All Started with Dance

Young or old, male or female, everyone dances. Infants and children delight in expressing themselves at almost any opportunity by moving to music. Teens, nervous about the idea of being held closely, will nonetheless dance with a new partner with reckless abandon at gatherings, parties and other social events. Adults also find considerable enjoyment in pairing with a partner and moving gracefully together as one. Dancing is always around and with us, providing pleasure, enjoyment, relaxation and exercise. It seems natural that something as universal as dance would not only be practiced, but studied and perfected. Not just as an art or science, but as a universal philosophical ideal.

Born in Japan, my parents carried me as an infant in their arms to local summer festivals. In mid-August these included Buddhist bon festivals with bon dances, in honor of the spirits of ancestors who, during three days, can return briefly to visit their families. The bon festivals commonly began and ended with a bonfire. The dance itself is a communal folk dance where individuals move in patterns unique to the local area, and, as a group, dance in a large circle around a scaffold to the beating of drums and the sounds of local folk songs. As a young child, I danced alongside my parents and copied their movements. As a preteen, I joined my friends in savoring the joy of Japanese social folk dancing. As a young adult, I regularly returned to my hometown to join my parents' adult neighbors, elevating such dancing to a spiritual experience. I was so inspired that I began evening ballroom and Latin dance lessons at City Hall in order to attend the more Western-style Christmas and holiday dances at my work. I learned basic waltz, tango, rumba, cha-cha and jitterbug, much to my parents' chagrin. This was post World War II, and Western dance was regarded by people of my parents' age as foreign and "loose"—indirectly "dancing with the enemy." While my colleagues and I liked our work parties with Western music and dance, in particular jitterbugging, partner dancing, unique to the West, was still publicly looked down upon in Japan.

When I moved to California, I met my future husband, Dan, at a YMCA dance. Dan was a "keen amateur," meaning he was studying American ballroom and Latin dance from professionals for performance and, ultimately, amateur competition.

We moved to Hawaii where, at the time, there were over 15 ballroom and Latin dance organizations, together serving roughly fifteen-thousand dancers, including about a hundred amateur competitors taking lessons from a multitude of professional dance instructors at professional dance studios. Amateur ballroom and Latin dancing were commonplace, and instruction proved both excellent and affordable.

The professional instructor working with Dan in Hawaii at that time, was searching for a competitive dance partner for him. Still speaking limited English, I ended up on the sidelines watching, occasionally filling in for this ideal future competition dance partner who had yet to be identified. It was during one such "stand in" moment that the professional paused, cocked an eyebrow, and announced she had found Dan's new competition dance partner: Me! Dan and I immediately began training as an amateur competitive dance couple.

After placing well in local and then state amateur American-style dance competitions, we were "discovered" by professional ten dance champion and coach, Mr. Albert Franz, and switched from the American to the International style of dance. To this day, we continue to work with Mr. Franz as well as other resident and any visiting amateur champions and professionals.

BALLROOM DANCE IN THE USA

Looking back, I've come to realize that this is where my later search for somatic therapy actually began. It may seem obtuse, but dance is probably one of the oldest forms of somatic therapy. It is where partners have touched and danced together socially for millennia. Ballroom dancing, on the other hand, is a more recent phenomena initiating within, and to some extent remaining within, high society.

Professional social dance masters first appeared in New York City around 1686 in order to teach manners to the children of the well-to-do. According to Richard M. Stephenson and Joseph Iaccarino in their book, *The Complete Book of Ballroom Dancing*, from the mid-1700s to the late-1800s there were seven dancing academies in the city. In the mid-nineteenth century, when Allen Dodworth opened his dance academy, he emphatically stated in his 1885 book *Dancing and its Relation to Education and Social Life: With a New Method of Instruction*, that dancing was not just for social amusement; its significance actually went much further—it dealt with "matters to do with men's souls." His book was in use for more than three decades and was considered one of the classics in its field. At the same time, Ward McAllister, another professional New York dance master, told socially ambitious New Yorkers that "social elevation" was the real reason for dance. Stephenson and Iaccarino state that McAllister offered ongoing family dance circle classes that were actually social parties by invitation only.

By 1900, rapid city growth suddenly brought vast numbers of immigrants and young people into the cities. With limited money, and no radio, television, movies, cars, cell phones or computers, young "good" men and women discovered public dance halls instead of bars and brothels. Social dance halls had served in smaller cities as centers for community activities. In larger cities, they were almost strictly commercial.

Stephenson and Iaccarino also mentioned that of the various types of commercial dance halls, there were also "bad" ones, like the taxi-dance halls or dime-a-dance establishments which flourished from the mid-nineteenth century through World War II.

"Hostesses" or "instructresses" provided instruction and a social dance for a fee, usually for less than a minute. Minute dances could, it was often assumed, lead to a more intimate relationship if all went well.

Vernon and Irene Castle

Social dance was given a tremendous boost just before World War I by Vernon and Irene Castle. Born in England, William Vernon Blyth came to New York in 1906 and began appearing on the vaudeville stage as a comic actor, magician, singer and dancer. He married vaudeville actress Irene Foote, and the two changed their names. Shortly thereafter, they went to Paris to take part in a musical show, "The Hen-Pecks," but the show lasted only a short time, and they turned, out of desperation, to exhibition dancing in cafes and restaurants. They were quickly befriended by "Papa Louis," owner of the Café de Paris who allowed them to give nightly exhibitions. After an outstanding year in Paris, they returned to New York City and soon became the most celebrated dance team in the world. Adopted by New York City society, they established Castle House as a studio for lessons in "refined" ballroom dancing to live music played by the Castle House Orchestra. In their book, *Modern Dancing*, they described the One-Step, Hesitation Waltz, tango and maxixe. They later established Castle Park at Coney Island "so that vacationing New Yorkers could keep up with their dance lessons." Soon the exclusive Castle Club and Castles-by-the-Sea were established. In

1914, the Castles appeared together in a musical named *Watch Your Step* with songs written especially for them by Irving Berlin. By 1915, they were performing regularly at Castles-in-the-Air, a roof-garden above the Forty-Fourth Street Theater, at the outrageous salary of $1,500 a week—American ballroom dancing had come of age.

Irene Castle distinguished between "afternoon tea" social dancing and "evening formal" ballroom dancing, in the process not only establishing a uniquely "American" dancing style, but also influencing dress in ballroom dancing. For example, she endorsed the elastic Castle Corset, recommending pleated petticoats with lace to hide the ankles, silk stockings with at most two pairs of garters, silk bloomers and a new French undergarment called a "brassiere." She was the first to popularize looseness in the sleeves to prevent binding when the arms were raised. Comfortable shoes, such as pumps, with a moderate heel held firmly in place with ribbons, completed a dance costume that would be not unfamiliar to ballroom dancers today.

Ballroom dancing as envisioned by Vernon and Irene was exclusive and expensive. It soon became both a sport and a signature of the wealthy and socially privileged.

Arthur Murray

In 1920, ballroom dancing took a new turn. A young dance teacher named Murray Techman, who later adopted the professional name of Arthur Murray, began offering inexpensive home dancing instruction by correspondence course. Stephenson and Iaccarino relate that eventually some five million Americans would register for home social dance lessons and learn the Arthur Murray method of ballroom dancing.

Arthur Murray began his dancing career in 1912, when he won a waltz contest at the age of 17. That same year, he invested two hundred dollars in dance lessons from Vernon and Irene Castle, afterward announcing himself publicly as a professional New York City dance teacher. Thirty years later, his business had grown to become a chain of franchised studios throughout the United States.

Fred Astaire and Ginger Rogers

According to Stephenson and Iaccarino, show dancer Fred Astaire got his big break in a movie called *Dancing Lady*. Later, in 1933, he and Ginger Rogers danced a tango and samba in the movie *Flying Down to Rio*. The following years, they starred and danced in *The Gay Divorcee* featuring Cole Porter's famous hit songs, "Night and Day" and "The Continental," then *Roberta* with the hit song "Smoke Gets in Your Eyes," *Top Hat* which included the all-time hit "Dancing Cheek to Cheek," followed by *Swing Time* and *Follow the Fleet*, capped by *The Story of Vernon and Irene Castle*. As a result of these movies and his growing popularity, the Fred Astaire method of ballroom dancing emerged. In 1936, it was estimated by Donald Grant, then president of the Dancing Teachers' Business Association, that because of the Castles, Arthur Murray, Fred Astaire and Ginger Rogers, six million people were learning social dance in various franchised studios across the USA.

THE IMPERIAL SOCIETY OF TEACHERS OF DANCING (ISTD)

While big American-franchised dance studios continued to train millions more dancers in their unique American figures and styles of dance, in 1924, the Ballroom Branch of the Imperial Society for Teachers of Dance, or ISTD, was founded in England to bring order to the world's ballroom dances, many of which had been developed in the USA and brought to Europe during World War I.

According to ISTD, the intent of this society was to codify, elaborate and "perfect" these dances. What resulted, however, was an "English," later known as the "International," style of ballroom dancing that would be taught from a single set of syllabi by dance teachers all over the world, the exception, of course, being the USA. ISTD selected the waltz, foxtrot, tango and quickstep, developing their own versions of these popular American dances based on natural walking movements. These so called "standard" dances were organized into syllabi with specific figures that were to be taught and mastered in a fixed order by academic fellows, dance masters and student teachers as well as their students. The dances themselves were further adjusted so they could be danced to popular tempos of music like ragtime and the Charleston.

John Lawrence Reynolds, in his book *Ballroom Dancing: The Romance, Rhythm and Style*, published in 1998, related that soon after organizing the "standard" dances, ISTD-qualified teachers began to similarly organize the various Latin-American dances. The idea behind standardized dance syllabi was that "correctly" trained dancers could dance with other "correctly" trained dancers anywhere in the world. What resulted, however, was that this influenced American studios to follow suit and categorize the various ballroom dances into a similar but wide variety of American styles, such as the Arthur Murray, Fred Astaire, Betty White and countless others styles all of which were later loosely organized into a variety of proficiency levels.

In response, there would eventually emerge one set of syllabi for social dancers and another "stricter" set for keen amateurs and future instructors being taught by ISTD teachers elsewhere in the world. International syllabi were reassembled into student teacher, associate, member and fellow proficiency levels.

America, isolated from the rest of the world, has as many different American styles, methods and syllabi as there are studios. What all the styles nowadays have in common is the idea of comprehensive proficiency levels for social, keen amateurs and competitors. On the other hand, ballroom dancing in the other nine-tenths of the world, led by ISTD, continued to maintain four and may soon host five different sets of proficiencies based on whether one is a social dancer, keen amateur, performer, competitor or DanceSport athlete.

THE BALLROOM DANCES

Waltz and Viennese Waltz

In their book, Stephenson and Iaccarino report that ballroom dancing probably started with the waltz, (from the German verb *waltzen* meaning to turn, roll or glide) born in the alpine regions of Austria and danced socially in the suburbs of Vienna.

The waltz as we know it today was supposedly danced for the first time in the USA in Boston in 1834 by Lorenzo Papanii, a Boston dance master, at a Beacon Hill socialite exhibition. Civic leaders who attended were generally insulted by what they called "an indecorous exhibition." As late as the mid-1800s, the waltz was still regarded by many as a wicked dance.

Beginning around 1830, Franz Lanner and Johann Strauss the younger introduced the Viennese Waltz, a faster version played at about 55-60 bars per minute. This led to development of the *valse a deux pas*, or the waltz with two steps danced to three beats of music. By 1900, a typical dance program was three quarters waltzes and one quarter all other dances combined.

In the late 1800s, two further modifications of the waltz developed in the United States. First was the Boston, a slow waltz with long gliding steps, fewer and slower turns, and more forward and backward movement, somewhat like the English Two-step. The second was the appearance of the waltz hesitations—the "One Step"—which involves taking one step to three beats of music.

Foxtrot and Quickstep

In *The History of Dance*, Mary Clarke and Clement Crisp describe the Cakewalk, a high-stepping African-American vaudeville dance popular in the late 1800s, replete with stylized costumes—a tall black hat, tall white collar, black coat and tails for men, and elaborate swirling frocks for women. On page 106 of their book, Clarke and Crisp say that, "brilliantly performed, it [the Cakewalk] acquired an almost theatrical flavor in its progress through the southern States to New York. From there it entered the ballrooms of society." The Cakewalk was a precursor to the foxtrot.

Stephenson and Iaccarino claim, however, that the foxtrot by name, was first danced in the Garden de Dance on the roof of the New York Theater. As part of an act downstairs, Harry Fox was doing trotting steps to ragtime music which people called "Fox's Trot." Wishing to capitalize on this, management introduced the dance with Cakewalk elegance upstairs.

The foxtrot is undoubtedly the most significant dance of all time in ballroom dancing. According to Stephenson and Iaccarino, its combination of quick and slow steps permitted more flexibility and greater dancing pleasure than the monotonous one and two-step dances which it quickly replaced. It is said that there is more variety in the foxtrot than in any other ballroom dance, and because of this, it is, technically speaking, the most difficult of ballroom dances to fully master.

Like waltz, two variations developed: a slower version,

danced at about 40 bars per minute and nicknamed the Peabody, and a faster one danced at over 50 bars per minute. The second version was particularly popular in England, where the ISTD in 1924 assigned it the name "quickstep," dictating that it be danced at 54 to 56 beats per minute. Clarke and Crisp note that the quickstep is actually a combination of "quick" foxtrot elements and the American Charleston.

Tango

The tango's origins, say Clarke and Crisp, lie deep in Argentine slave dancing, the slaves having come from Africa by way of Cuba. Reynolds states that by the late nineteenth century, "tango," probably meaning "touch," had become popular in the slums of Buenos Aires, where dancers in the barrios called it *barrios con corte*, or "slum dance with a rest," referring to the manner in which the dancers would suddenly pause for a beat or two before resuming.

Early tango music and dance were widely regarded as obscene. Many tangos are indeed scandalous, some are still written for and danced by prostitutes to show off their wares to prospective clients.

In the USA, it was the Castles along with Hollywood superstar Rudolf Valentino who popularized tango with its various sexually suggestive moves, and, according to Reynolds, introduced it to American dancers. Clarke and Crisp note that its popularity was such that in London, where many learned it from

Gladys Crozier's book *The Tango and How to Dance It*, there emerged popular "Tango Teas" held in the afternoons at the most fashionable hotels.

In Europe, tango was later reduced by the ISTD to a series of quick motions of the dancers' heads and staccato foot motions, eliminating the intimate sexualized moves and caresses. According to Reynolds, ballroom tango today exists in three distinct forms: the International Ballroom, American Smooth and Argentine versions.

By the 1930s, as Clarke and Crisp state, the "Standard Four" dances—the waltz, foxtrot, quickstep and tango—were being danced everywhere in the world in the International style, except in America where Americans were continuing to evolve ever more versions of the American smooth dances, today comprising primarily waltz, Viennese Waltz, foxtrot and tango.

THE LATIN DANCES

Rumba

If ballroom dances appealed to the older population, then Latin dances appealed to both old and young. According to Stephenson and Iaccarino, the true rumba is of African origin, and like the tango, was danced primarily by the lowest strata of society because of the licentious character of the dance. On page 43 of *The Complete Book of Ballroom Dancing*, they relate that "the native rumba folk dance is essentially a sex pantomime danced extremely fast with exaggerated hip movements and with a sensually aggressive attitude on the part of the man and a defensive attitude on the part of the woman."

During the Second World War, the Son, a "cleaned up" version of the rumba, became popular with middle class dancers in Cuba, and with it, rumba was transfigured from a dance of sex to "The Dance of Love."

In the late 1920s, Xavier Cugat introduced "American rumba" to the USA at the famed Coconut Grove in Los Angeles. Soon after, it appeared in the early sound movie, In *Gay Madrid*, and a distinctively American version was introduced by Cugat to eager dancers at the Waldorf-Astoria Hotel in New York.

The American rumba, note Stephenson and Iaccarino, is a direct modification of the Son, and in some instances, it is still called by that name. In the American style it is danced in a box pattern similar to the Bronze (first) level American Waltz but with three steps to four beats of music. Its chief characteristic is "Cuban motion," a discreet but expressive hip movement achieved by carefully timed weight transfer from side to side. English rumba is danced differently, substituting distinctive forward-and-back steps supposedly to de-emphasize the sexually-evocative Cuban motion.

Mambo

In the back country of Haiti, the mambo was primarily a voodoo dance. Researching the dance, Stephenson and Iaccarino came to the conclusion, "there is no folk dance in Haiti called the 'Mambo'."

The above authors also state that mambo, as we know it today, is attributable to Perez Prado, who introduced an Americanized version to visiting Americans at La Tropicana nightclub in Havana in 1943. Initially that dance included violent acrobatics. "Ballroom mambo" appeared almost simultaneously at dance studios, resort hotels and at nightclubs throughout New York and Miami, though initially it was mostly of artistic and commercial interest. However, when Rosemary Clooney sang "Mambo Italiano" and Nat King Cole "Papa Loves Mambo," mambo became the newest Latin dance rage.

Stephenson and Iaccarino further relate that, in England, where rumba and mambo are danced with a quick-quick-slow forward-and-back basic motion the mambo was considered a modification of the rumba and eventually dropped. In the United States, where the box-style rumba basic is still widely danced, dance teachers typically regard the mambo as a unique dance and include it in American Latin dance competitions.

Cha-Cha

Even at its peak of popularity, many dancers did not seem to care for the mambo. In particular, many ballroom dancers criticized the fast mambo for having more of the jerky character of social jitterbug and none of the smooth movements usually associated with refined Latin dance. Stephenson and Iaccarino relate that many especially found the pause on the first beat with syncopated foot movements roughly on the 2-3-4 to be unnatural. In 1953, a Cuban orchestra named "America" played mambo with a slight triple step undulation on the fourth or slow count and, *voilà*, the cha-cha was born. By 1959, dance studios reported it to be the single most popular ballroom and Latin dance in America, which it remains to this day.

Most ballroom dancers, American and International, are more comfortable with the cha-cha and samba (with its variety of seven different rhythms, one of which is, in fact, a cha-cha time rhythm) than with mambo's inherently unusual rhythm. Also, cha-cha lends itself easily to quick dramatic styling variations.

Samba

According to Stephenson and Iaccarino, two Brazilian folk dances made their way early into the American and Latin ballroom: the maxixe and the samba. Starting about 1910, the maxixe, or Tango Bresilien, was one of three "classic" dances greatly favored by the Castles; however, while an excellent interpretive performance dance, it was danced more like a tango and proved difficult for social dancers to learn and enjoy.

Samba or *carioca* (technically "rocking samba") was widely danced by Brazilians partying in downtown Rio de Janeiro on holidays and at Rio Carnival. It was an easy dance to learn, according to Stephenson and Iaccarino, exuding high energy and considerable sexual power. During Rio Carnival, "schools of *carioca*" dance samba in long processions involving thousands of elaborately costumed dancers interpreting various national themes danced to popular Brazilian music. The dance was introduced to United States movie audiences in 1933 by Fred Astaire and Dolores Del Rio when they danced the *carioca* in *Flying Down to Rio*. Several years later, it was reintroduced by Carmen Miranda in *That Night in Rio*.

The samba is a moderately popular ballroom dance, limited to advanced ballroom dancers mainly because of its speed, and seven different rhythms. Characteristics of contemporary samba include rapid "cuts" or steps taken on syncopated quarter beats and a pronounced whole body rocking motion and sway.

Paso Doble

Paso doble, the fourth contemporary Latin dance, is danced to characteristic two-beat march music, traditionally part of the procession at the beginning of a bullfight. In fact, paso doble literally means "two-step." Clarke and Crisp relate that paso doble, with its many reflections of bullfighting, is Spanish in origin, but was refined for the ballroom by French dance masters. It is primarily an "exhibition" dance in which the man represents the matador and the woman his cape (not the bull as is often claimed). Usually the last of the classical competitive International-style Latin dances to be learned, it is rarely danced in amateur circles due to the high skill-level required to make it attractive to judges and audiences alike.

East Coast Swing and Jive

On March 12, 1926, when the Savoy Ballroom opened its doors in New York City, its first act featured an impressive block-long dance floor with a raised double bandstand. Consistently providing the best in fast swing-jazz music of the day, Stephenson and Iacarrino report that dancers developed a colloquial, athletic, often highly acrobatic form applicable to almost any emerging musical variation so long as it had "that swing." Swing, on the other hand, was not so easily defined, though it loosely meant a subtle pulsation in 4/4 or common time.

In 1927, following Charles Lindbergh's flight to Paris, a local dancer named "Shorty George" Snowden is said to have referred to the dance as "Lindy's Hop." Today, the Lindy Hop, or just Lindy, also known as swing, jitterbug, rock 'n' roll and jive is still highly popular at American social and ballroom dances. Lindy is currently danced in two syncopated two-step chassés accenting the offbeat and followed by a break or back step, recognized as the characteristic feature of the dance. By the end of 1936, the Lindy swept the United States. Under one of its most popular names, "jitterbug," it rapidly became an American pastime. With the entry of the United States into the Second World War, Clarke and Crisp noted it spread like wildfire to every part of the world eventually acquiring the name, "East Coast Swing," its formal American Latin name. It was subsequently reinterpreted in England by ISTD into the more rigorous and upbeat International Jive.

DANCE SYLLABI AND STYLES

USA DanceSport, the part of USA Dance (formerly the United States Amateur Ballroom Dancers Association or US-ABDA, currently USADance) that administers amateur DanceSport, the competitive discipline of ballroom and Latin dancing, defined a syllabus in the *2002 USA DanceSport Rules* as a "list of fundamental dance figures, organized by style, dance and professional level."

ISTD

In the early 1920s, Philip Richardson, then editor of *The Dancing Times*, called a series of informal conferences of teachers of ballroom dancing to bring order to the increasing number of emerging styles of ballroom and Latin dance. As a result, in 1924, ISTD officially created a ballroom branch and five ISTD dance teachers were chosen to write a single, internationally-recognized list of "syllabus steps." The committee, according to Clarke and Crisp, included Josephine Bradley, Eve Tynegate-Smith, Muriel Simmons, Leslie Humphreys and Victor Silvester. Basically, the committee reviewed and then reinterpreted for the British (and thereby for all the world's dancers), a single style and method of dance figures based on "natural walking movement" with the feet parallel and the man leading the woman in close embrace (the man typically moving forward and his partner moving backward), directing her progress across the ballroom floor. The committee eventually worked out syllabi for the teaching of four "standard" (now called "ballroom") dances: the waltz, foxtrot, tango and quickstep, which have since been taught in the same way by ISTD-certified dance teachers throughout the world. Known collectively as "International-style" ballroom dances, the emphasis was to correctly maintain the rhythm, timing and footwork of each individual dance at "lower" proficiency levels, adding technique, musicality and expressive performance at "higher" proficiency levels. To these four standard International ballroom dances was later added the "modern" Viennese Waltz, and later, five International-style Latin-American dances: the rumba, cha-cha, samba, paso doble and jive.

It eventually fell upon Alex Moore, considered by many ISTD committee members as the foremost authority on International ballroom technique, the first Chairperson of the International Council of Ballroom Dancing and author of the 1936 classic, *Ballroom Dancing*, and its 1954 sequel, *Popular Variations*, to further refine the styling techniques. In 1971, Sidney Francis, Doris Lavelle, Doris Nichols, Dimitri Petrides, Elizabeth Romain and Peggy Spencer would be called upon to similarly formalize the International style of Latin-American dance through the publication of *The Revised Technique of Latin-American Dancing*.

International ballroom (formerly standard) dances are referred to as such to distinguish them from the many different American Smooth Style dances, the roots of which remained within the major U.S. studio chains following in the footsteps of Arthur Murray and Fred Astaire. Reynolds points out that American styles, in the tradition of Astaire in his popular movies, encourage frequent breaks from the closed position, permitting the partners to improvise and dance without any physical contact between them, a feature International-style dancers point to as a characteristic of the Latin-American dances.

Arthur Murray and the American Style

In the 1958 version of his book, *Murray-Go-Round*, Arthur Murray explains, "After 25 years of teaching, I hit upon a discovery that changed our entire system of teaching. I found that one easy step was the basis for 75% of all existing Fox-Trot steps. We call it the Magic Step...because it can be done in 27 different ways." This pattern, based on two slow and two quick steps, is the foundation for the Arthur Murray style and syllabi.

In 1938, Arthur Murray, in his book *How to Become a Good Dancer*, published the first American-style syllabi; it included American Waltz (13 figures), foxtrot (8 figures), tango (5 figures), rumba (6 figures), cha-cha (4 figures), mambo (6 figures), merengue (5 figures), samba (7 figures), swing (5 figures) and rock 'n' roll (4 figures). Figures were accompanied by rhythm, timing, foot positions, alignment, turn, rise and fall, poise, hold and sway with limited information on foot rise, foot work (the part of the foot in contact with the floor) and floor craft. In the case of foxtrot, it also included a basic amalgamated routine. Later in his 1953 book, *Let's Dance*, he briefly introduced the concepts of interpretation and variation. Note that the American style included merengue and rock 'n' roll, both of which are still included in the Arthur Murray American-style dances, and are popular nightclub dances.

Fred Astaire and the American Style

The Fred Astaire syllabi, first published in 1962 in *The Fred Astaire Dance Book*, were written specifically to explain and promote "the Fred Astaire Dance Studio Method." In the book, Astaire lists the American Waltz (9 figures), foxtrot (7 figures), tango (9 figures), polka (5 figures), the "Fred Astaire Swing Trot" (5 figures), rumba (9 figures), mambo (7 figures), cha-cha (8 figures), samba (7 figures), Lindy Swing (6 figures) and the twist ("simple basic" only). Figures were accompanied by rhythm, timing, foot position, foot rise, foot work, turn, poise, hold, sway and included select performance amalgamations and basic demonstration routines. The 1978 version added body movement, including "contrary body movement" and "continuity styling," both further emphasizing the quality of movement. Perhaps because of its attention to detail, the Fred Astaire American style is still today often referred to simply as "The American Style." Both the Arthur Murray and Fred Astaire American-style syllabi, as originally published, included only one basic proficiency level.

ISTD and USISTD's American Style

In actuality, there were, and still are, as many American

"styles" and syllabi as there are major studios. Each has its own particular names, descriptions, methods, techniques, characteristics and approaches to ballroom dancing. Perhaps it was the existence of these many American styles, each with general absence of proficiency levels, that led the ISTD to later tentatively define a set of American-style teacher syllabi at three proficiency levels, namely, student teacher, associate and licentiate. Teachers could then introduce proficiency-appropriate groupings of figures to social dancers, logically-graduated figures and amalgamations to Keen Amateurs, and test and present proficiency medals to those who want "outside" certification of their proficiency as they progressed through Bronze, Silver and Gold levels. At the same time, American franchise studios were developing and spreading their own similar proficiency tasks and levels.

As of 2005, the ISTD American-style syllabi includes waltz, (20 figures with 7 variations), foxtrot (22 figures with 4 variations), tango (19 figures), Viennese Waltz (20 figures), Peabody (19 figures), rumba (20 figures), mambo (20 figures), cha-cha (20 figures), swing (22 figures) and bolero (20 figures), including aspects of dance only partially addressed in Arthur Murray or Fred Astaire syllabi. But do these syllabi actually reflect the emerging American style? Despite ISTD's formation of an American branch, the USISTD, and the extent of the USISTD American-style syllabi, I think not. Furthermore, I think this opinion is reflected in various statements by USA Dance, recognized as the sole certifying body for amateur DanceSport in the USA by the National Governing Body for DanceSport, the

United States Olympic Committee and the International DanceSport Federation. In the end, what can be said is that while the International-style ballroom and Latin-American figures have been codified into a single, consistent set of syllabi recognized throughout 90% of the world, the many American-style Smooth and Rhythm syllabi differ significantly depending on the organization supporting them. Currently, the majority of American-style competitors compete in America within proficiency levels. Despite the existence of Bronze, Silver, Gold, Gold Star, Gold Bar and others, American-style syllabi and proficiency levels as presently devised are insufficient to wholly support or represent American style in the emerging world of DanceSport. This is quite different from International-style competition where competitors compete within Pre-novice, Novice, Pre-Championship and Championship levels which correspond directly with emerging world DanceSport proficiency levels.

USA Dance and the National Dance Council of America's American Style

USA Dance, formerly the United States Amateur Ballroom Dancers Association or USABDA, as of 2005 recognized the following American-style syllabi organized into Pre-Bronze, Bronze and Silver proficiency levels, Gold being essentially any figures not otherwise specified: waltz (22 figures), foxtrot (28 figures), tango (20 figures), Viennese Waltz (20 figures), Peabody (10 figures), rumba (25 figures), mambo (22 figures), cha-cha (20 figures), East Coast Swing (22 figures) and bolero (20 figures). Up to 2004, certification by USA Dance (USABDA) was required of all amateur competitors dancing for the USA, giving these particular syllabi considerable weight in the competitive world.

Near this same time, the National Dance Council of America (NDCA), the recognized certifying body for professionals split with USA Dance over control of amateur competition and published its own American-style syllabi, similar to USA Dance's American-style syllabi but onerously including over 100 prohibited figures, steps and actions at the Novice proficiency level.

American and International Style Olympic DanceSport

DanceSport, as it is called today, was first recognized by the United States and International Olympic Committees as an international athletic competitive sport in 1989. Peter Pover, then President of the United States Amateur Ballroom Dancers Association (currently USA Dance), in an article entitled "What is DanceSport?" published in the January/February 1999 edition of *Amateur Dancer* (now *American Dancer*), defined DanceSport, (including dancesport or dance sport) as any and all forms of athletic dance commonly referred to as smooth and rhythm dancing in the USA, and as standard/ballroom and Latin-American dancing internationally, that require specialized athletic knowledge, discipline and muscle development to perform. Put more simply, DanceSport is competitive smooth/standard/ballroom and rhythm/Latin-American partner dance.

DanceSport, Pover points out, is now divided into two divisions: ballroom (waltz, foxtrot, tango, quickstep and Viennese Waltz) and Latin-American (rumba, cha-cha, samba, paso doble, and jive), loosely following the ISTD International style of competitive dance. Since there are two different world dance styles, International and American, either is permitted (this is sometimes called "open" competition versus closed or syllabi-restricted competition). Pre-Olympic proficiency levels include Pre-novice, Novice, Pre-championship and Championship. Hopeful couples begin as Pre-Novices and must progress through each proficiency level by accumulating five "points" for placing in top positions in sanctioned events with a semi-final round at local, regional and national DanceSport competitions. While DanceSport, like all Olympic events, is by definition restricted to amateurs, DanceSport is currently danced in Amateur, Amateur-Professional (Pro-Am) and Professional categories. According to the *2002/3 USA DanceSport Rule Book* (online), USA Dance is the officially recognized certifying body for amateur competitors—called USA DanceSport Athletes—as distinguished from the National Dance Council of America (NDCA), which is the primary certifying body for professional competitors.

Pover mentions in his 1999 article that the International DanceSport Federation (IDSF) was formed in 1957 to organize member associations further at the national and world level. IDSF, in turn, recognized USA Dance as the sole certifying body for amateur competitors representing USA in world DanceSport events. USA Dance in return created the United States Dance

Sport Council (USDSC) which issued the first official USA DanceSport rule book. Under the rules of the IDSF and USDSC, a recognized DanceSport competition is one that is officially sanctioned by a member organization of the IDSF and/or World Dance and Dance Sport Council (WD&DSC is the officially recognized International Sports Federation for Professionals). This means that competitors at USA DanceSport National, Regional and Chapter Championships as well as any other USA DanceSport sanctioned competitions and any NDCA Recognized Competitions accrue proficiency points towards Olympic and World DanceSport Competition.

An interesting historical aside was made by Ann Rodrigues in her article entitled "Ice Dance and DanceSport" in the May/June 1998 *Amateur Dancers* magazine, that DanceSport was originally envisioned as analogous to Ice Dance, an established Winter Olympic event since 1976. Ice dancers use the basic elements of figure skating—use of edges, stroking, speed, smooth turns—as well as the principles of good dancing—posture, balance, partnering skill and fluid motion—to create a choreographed dance on ice with artistic beauty that captures the essence of a particular dance. It's not an accident that some early DanceSport teachers taught Olympic ice skaters how to dance on ice and were largely responsible for creating Ice Dance, considered by many to be one of the most watched Olympic events. As Reynolds stated on page 156 of his book, *Ballroom Dancing*, DanceSport "draw[s] attention to dancing's superb role model of compromise, cooperation, and mutual respect."

Rodrigues further points out that DanceSport athletes, like Olympic ice dancers, must develop both general and specific athletic abilities through rigorous training. Both must perform memorized groups of basic figures as well as respect their partnership and interpret the music in a way that pleases both judges and audiences. Both DanceSport and Olympic ice dancing involve both male and female athletes working together as one— most other Olympic sports and dance forms aren't partnered or as gender-equitable. As a final aside, DanceSport competitions are judged by the Skating System rather than by reference to any specific syllabi.

About 20 years ago in the USA, states began including "ballroom dancing" as an amateur competitive sport in pre-Olympic games—for example, the Aloha State Games in Hawaii. The ballroom dancing competition portion of the games, the largest and most popular multi-sport competition in Hawaii, began June 13, 1998, and was hosted by USA Dance Honolulu (formerly USABDA Honolulu). According to Mr. Roger Izumigawa, former Commissioner of DanceSport for the Pacific Region, ballroom dancing as a pre-Olympic competitive event has been successfully received with spectators and competitors alike being treated like Olympic attendees.

By public demand, the International Olympic Committee (IOC) agreed to pre-trial DanceSport as a potential Olympic event by scheduling a DanceSport Exhibition in the 2000 Olympics Closing Ceremony and the 2002 Olympic Arts Festival held continuously throughout the 2002 Olympic and Paralympic Winter Games. Although there currently remains no room for any new Olympic events, the International World Games Association (IWGA) agreed to designate DanceSport as a World Game at the request of IOC. World Games are held to honor sports that have full recognition by IOC but are awaiting a slot in the Olympic program. The Sixth World Games, held August 25 and 26, 2001, in Akita, Japan, included both ballroom and Latin-American DanceSport competitions. Competitors represented 28 of the 73 countries participating in the World Olympics. DanceSport has become a regular event in the World Games, held every four years, since 1997, including more recently, the 2005 World Games in Duisburg, Germany, the 2009 World Games in Kaohsuing, Chinese Taipei and the 2013 World Games in Cali, Colombia. World Games are currently scheduled in 2017 in Wroclaw, Poland and 2021 in Birmingham, Alabama, USA.

The major effect of pre-Olympic DanceSport has been to redefine competition, moving it away from any particular syllabus style. At present, although organized along the lines of the ISTD International style, USA DanceSport has stated that "basic" figures need be neither defined nor compulsory. Sanctioned DanceSport competitions generally reflect this by emphasizing "Open" competition and the use of the Skating System for judging.

International Versus American-style DanceSport

Syllabus differences between the various American and International styles of ballroom dance have already been mentioned. For example, American Style Smooth and Rhythm syllabi include different dances, dance figures, methods, approaches and techniques than International ballroom and Latin-American syllabi at social, keen amateur and beginning competitor levels.

More fundamentally, however, International-style ballroom dances are generally danced in a highly stylized, closed position, addressing both posture and frame, with the lady's right hand in the gentleman's left, her left hand on his right shoulder and his right hand on her shoulder blade, or, in the case of tango, on her lower back. This creates a single vertical center of balance that each partner uses in his or her movements. American-style smooth dances are danced in open, semi-closed and closed position, with the dancers generally maintaining separate centers of weight and balance.

Differences can also be noted between American-style rhythm and International-style Latin-American syllabi, but most top-level DanceSport teachers, coaches and dancers will say that to be successful in DanceSport, one must ultimately incorporate and demonstrate elements of each.

Chapter 2
The Language of Dance

The previous chapter was focused mainly on couple's social dance to DanceSport, including performance and competition, with emphasis on the definitions; history; dance criteria; International and American styles; open events; differences between amateur, pro-am and professional competition; categories (for example, age); and the gradual development of World Olympic DanceSport. Some important somatic elements of dance emerged and been identified: posture; balance; partnering skills; fluid [rhythmic] motion; partnership compromise, cooperation, and mutual respect; and touch. In subsequent chapters, these will become important focus elements in the development of a definition of somatic therapy. In this second chapter, I would like to move the focus almost exclusively from performance to the underlying creative process in dance, especially DanceSport, emphasizing and exploring the various methods of documenting these movements, referred to when prescribed as choreography, or, in other words, basic physical movements.

CHOREOGRAPHY

Webster's Seventh New College Dictionary defines choreography as the art of representing dance symbolically with a focus on composition and arrangement of dance figures. The attraction of today's DanceSport comes not so much from dancing precisely prescripted individual or group patterns, but rather from two people, traditionally, but not necessarily exclusively a male and female, dancing as one. Formation team ballroom performance and competition is probably the last precursor to modern DanceSport in which traditional ideas of choreography and dance notation are fully applicable.

Ellen Jacob, in *Dancing - A Guide for the Dancer You Can Be*, points out that in modern, jazz and stage dance, a professional choreographer usually acts as the "designer" of the dance; in DanceSport only professionals and the most successful amateur championship-level competitors routinely utilize a professional choreographer. It is important to remember that in the formal DanceSport world strict distinction is made between professional and amateur DanceSport based not on proficiency but on whether the dancers accept money for their dancing. DanceSport choreographers, Jacob states, are therefore commonly teachers or coaches who work holistically with a competitive couple in the short-term to highlight their strengths and in the long-term strengthen their weaknesses. In fact, based on the popular television series, "Dancing with the Stars," DanceSport choreography appears to be diverging from rather than converging towards mainstream choreographic perceptions and notation. This trend can be expected to continue well into the immediate and perhaps even well into the distant future.

THE CREATIVE PROCESS

It seems natural to assume that the creative process or more exactly, creative processes, involved in ballet, modern and jazz dance as well as DanceSport would be the same. Unfortunately, just as the definition of choreography depends to some extent on the form or kind of dance, so do the creative processes involved, even though ultimately, all are dances in their own right.

Dance

The eleventh edition of Merriam-Webster's Collegiate Dictionary defines dance as a rhythmic and patterned succession of bodily movements, usually performed to music. In other words, dance involves movement, rhythm, structure (groups of movements that together have meaning to the choreographer, dancer and/or viewer) and in almost all performance or competitive situations, music. I believe it necessary to regard dance as both a foundation and extension of music.

Music

Maurice Emmanuel, a Doctor of Arts and Doctor Laureate

of the Paris Conservatory of Dance, explains in his book, *The Antique Greek Dance*, that to the ancient Greeks, the ancestors of Western culture, music was a gift of the Muses (inspiration), as well as an art and science incorporating intelligible combinations of tones into a whole that has timing, rhythm, melody, harmony, structure and continuity. That is to say, to the Greeks, dance was inseparable from music. Clarke and Crisp further note that dance and music share at least two attributes, namely rhythm and structure, to which I would add timing, while dance adds to music the bodily expression of all the aforementioned attributes. The creative processes involved in any movement study should therefore reflect, at the least, musical timing, rhythm and structure, as well as corresponding bodily movements.

DanceSport Movement and Structure

As mentioned previously, amateur DanceSport performers and competitors commonly acquire instruction in fundamental DanceSport through study and acquisition of figures unique to each dance, techniques for interpretive expression, and the weaving of them together into each of the ten particular genres of DanceSport music using a multitalented coach rather than a choreographic specialist. Jacob alludes to this when she says that private classes best serve advanced students, professional dancers who need to develop audition material, and future dance teachers, while coaching is reserved for dancers who are preparing for a role in competitive DanceSport. DanceSport is, by default, both a performing and competitive athletic sport that in terms of viewer appeal in my opinion, expresses and explores male-female (or at least partnership) roles and relationships within particular musical genres and socio-cultural venues.

A significant difference between competitive DanceSport, which I practice, and modern, jazz, ballet and stage dance is that DanceSport competitors, in general, are permitted to choose the musical genre but not the particular musical piece they will dance to. For this reason, International DanceSport Adjudicator and former Organizer of the Hawaii Star Ball, Mr. Geoffrey Fells, stated in a 10 June 1997 communiqué to the author that DanceSport choreography emphasizes creation of groups of amalgamated figures, called routines, that can be effectively danced in competition to any musical piece within a particular musical genre.

It is common in modern, jazz, ballet or staged dance for the creative process to come from and be developed by a professional choreographer who, like a producer, chooses the music, figures and dancers, and then, like a movie director, weaves everything, including the individual dancers, together into a coherent composition spanning an entire musical production. In short, the product is built to progressively approach what the choreographer envisions as the final product. DanceSport routines on the other hand, evolve first from the figures which a couple does well together within a particular competitive musical genre, which dancers and coach together amalgamate using expressive movements called techniques as well as the music of the genre likely to be actually played, the conditions of the competition "stage" (e.g. the condition of the floor, the skill levels and the number of couples on the floor) and the number of competitive rounds that the couple will likely have to dance. Unlike performance, during actual competition all these elements are not fully under competitor or coach control. In social dance, they are moderately constrained, but couples are free to otherwise interpret and dance as they please, adding relaxed "fun" and "enjoyment" to the activity.

All types of dance, but especially DanceSport, generally begin with the dancers exploring their own native movements and qualities, all in terms of what *viewers* see rather than what the dancer feels at any moment. Unlike modern, jazz, ballet and staged dance, DanceSport, as well as social dance, is built almost exclusively on natural body movements, so, DanceSport routines, for me, usually begin with observing my own body movements in mirrors as I listen and naturally walk (Standard) or move my hip and torso (Latin-American) to a particular genre of music.

To paraphrase Jacob about the natural DanceSport creative process: Do you enjoy sustained, smooth-flowing motions or sharp, abrupt motions? Are your movements heavy and forceful or light and delicate? Do you feel rooted to the ground or like you are flying through space and time? Do you seem to make broad, sweeping gestures or move on a smaller, more contained scale? Are you suddenly doing tic movements with complex rhythms or sticking to simple shapes and figures? Which body parts do you isolate and which seem to move naturally to music?

To these, I must add that each partner must also constantly observe each other both separately and together: What do we, as a couple, naturally do in common?

After a practice dance, performance or competition we often talk together, discussing for hours what we can best do together and how it will look to the judges and audience.

Furthermore, modern, jazz, ballet and stage dancers do not commonly perform or compete in specialized male-female partnerships using close, closed hold frame. For this reason alone, DanceSport movements, routines, choreography and notation differ considerably from their analogs in modern and classical dance.

Finally, with DanceSport (as with Ice Dance), couples compete against each other before judges and an audience using the Skating System: Those couples that attract attention while executing a particular figure, movement or movement complex which they are particularly good at score higher. It is not as important to command constant attention and dance a totally cohesive dance, but rather to constantly convey the impression of good dancing, while inviting the attention of judges and audience at key "highlight" moments that show the partnership at its best. As such, routines in DanceSport commonly consist of dance phrases that demonstrate basic (sometimes called "compulsory," though they are not strictly compulsory) figures, interspersed with short, unexpected, unusual, visibly attractive movements of the body (or for that matter, costume), called variations, sometimes breaking stride, rhythm or even pausing in a photographic opportunity pose. The objective in DanceSport is not to be consistent in all parts of a prescripted grouping, but to interweave the expected with the unexpected in a unique way that focuses attention on one's partnership abilities at the most opportune moments. Hence, the very reason behind the choreographic coaching in competitive DanceSport is quite different from other forms of dance.

I would now like to focus on some of the elements of International-style competitive DanceSport that make creation of a competitive routine, coaching and execution in DanceSport competition or performance particularly interesting to me as a competitive dancer, a massage therapist and a somatic therapist.

International-Style Competition DanceSport Routines

First and foremost, partners typically work hard to show off the female, or in some cases, the following partner's flexibility and suppleness. Men (or in some instances, leaders or initiators) are expected to at the least, have the appearance of leading the other. Initiators have a considerable amount of intellectual as well as kinesthetic material to acquire. This is especially true early in one's training, in order to know how to signal a particular figure or phrase to enable the other partner to complete the figure or phrase and showcase it within the couple's particular expressive interpretative framework.

Women or the follower in any figure or phrase, like myself, must develop the strength and stamina to allow the man's power and control to be fully and seamlessly expressed by moving and building on his initial power movements, allowing them to visibly course through the body using key skills often referred to in DanceSport as connection and follow-through. In DanceSport, both partners initially learn and practice the mirror image basic dance skills and figures. Later, they incorporate increasingly specialized roles while always appearing as if the two are dancing as one. Ballet is possibly the only other dance form which assigns such highly specific movements to each sex or partner, according to Jacob. DanceSport movements are not strictly visual or rhythmic; they are instead highly kinesthetic while, to some extent at least, incorporating individual (some would say partnership) intuition during competitive execution. Highly kinesthetic or intuitive learning works well with natural movements that have an organic flow of their own—like the natural walking movement that is the very heart of social as well as DanceSport.

My primary coach, USA Ten Dance Champion and International DanceSport Adjudicator, Albert Franz, said during a coaching session that in competitive DanceSport, improvement requires being aware of movement details and slowly eliminating or replacing those that do not enhance the couple's natural movement appearance with ones that do. In DanceSport competition or performance, viewers do not know what the dancers actually feel kinesthetically, they only know what they imagine they feel. For this reason, I not only use coaching but practice my own part individually and together with my partner as often as I can while watching myself in mirrors. Even so, my partner and I try to cultivate a common or complementary inner feeling and emotion, knowing that it is from these inner feelings that the transcendent nature of dance will emerge and become appreciated by the audience. Mr. Franz often reminds me that no one wants to know how achy I really feel, only that I look like I am moving in intercourse with the music, my partner and the audience's imagination.

Dancing in closed, close frame brings up special issues of individual differences in physique, natural timing and movement quality. For example, I am only five feet tall, while my partner is five feet six inches tall. I have short arms, nearly the same length as my legs; he has long arms and short legs. My partner has a particularly broad chest that creates a wide, strong-appearing frame that is challenging for me to fit within, given my petite physique. Yet again, people often say my partner has natural rhythm, while for me, Western rhythms have never felt natural. Instead, I've had to work hard and learn to let go when my partner suddenly introduces a new syncopated Western variation into a routine I had memorized. Finally, my partner likes to make broad, sweeping movements involving lots of extension, whereas I tend to enjoy minute precision. On the other hand, my partner has trouble memorizing complex routines, while I don't at all. In short, he loves surprise and variation, while I love perfectly executing a movement exactly as I have memorized it in rehearsal. In DanceSport competition, however, we are judged on how well we not only perform individually and together, but how well we appear to do what we do as one. When we are successful, we invariably want a record of our movements so that we can do them again. The same could be said about any successful somatic maneuver.

DANCE NOTATION

Ever since people began dancing they have sought to record their movements, first in oral form, later in pictograms and finally writing. These records are a way to preserve a particular dance and allow one to reproduce it at will. This, and perhaps a desire to record a particularly impressive dance for posterity and take one's place in immortality, eventually led to the development of various styles of dance notation.

Ancient Greece

Maurice Emmanuel, a Doctor of Letters and a laureate of the Paris Conservatory of Dance, on pages ix-x of his classic 1916 book, *The Antique Greek Dance*, says, "The special qualities of Greek dance are a very keen sense of mimetic value, joined to perfect rhythm but somewhat lacking in precision"—not a bad definition of modern DanceSport. According to Emmanuel, the sixth century B.C. Greeks were fascinated, even obsessed, with representing the most memorable moments of their lives, whether a battle, funeral, sexual encounter or any other event through dance.

Today, we have come to realize that Greek pictographs,

paintings, even sculptures are more than static memorials. They are more accurately, multidimensional representations of actual dances, the "fourth dimension" being exquisite and detailed recordings of their dance movements through space and time. All that's been missing is a Rosetta stone for Greek music—a musical "key" that would allow us to recreate the music and then their dances in their entirety. Emmanuel relates on page xiii that for hundreds of years, Greek dance figures were always "stylistically" represented advancing on the left leg. Only recently have we become aware that this is a notational convention which allowed Greek artisans to "fix the fleeting 'moment' of a movement" such that, when recombined with the music, actually captured and recorded the dance in a series of pictographs not unlike a series of modern pictures in a video.

In ancient Greece, prizes were awarded at "dance games" in which dancers attempted to mimic life events with whole body movements synchronized to music, producing what they called eurythmy, which they valued more than anything else in dance. These dances incorporated leaping, running, throwing, stretching and other movements representing individual combat in the Pyrrhic dances to special moments of beauty, love, sexuality or worship. Such "dance games" closely parallel modern DanceSport competition (or one could contend, *vice versa*). Yet, Greek dance was more than "dance games" or simple eurythmy.

Emmanuel says on page xx, "the Greeks attached a wide significance to the word 'dance.' Every movement executed to [auditory or, for that matter internal] music was considered a dance." Common Greek dance movements were in fact, based on natural, later stylized body movements, much like today's social and competitive dance and now DanceSport. Interestingly, while Greek dance is distinctly whole-body in nature, its pictographic notation placed primary emphasis on foot position and foot movements. As Clarke and Crisp stated, figures and floor patterns are two of the most basic dance elements denoted in ancient as well as modern functional choreography.

Western Europe

Clarke and Crisp noted that in the 1700s, Raoul Feuillet, in his European dance notation book entitled, *Choreqraphie, ou l'art de decrire la danse*, provided the first guidebook for recording and reconstructing European period dances. According to Clarke and Crisp, *Stenochoregraphie*, by Arthur Saint-Leon and published in 1852, used pin figures above the top line of each musical stave to represent physical movements of the dancers. Alternatively, George Bickham, Jr., in his book, *An Easy Introduction to Dancing, or the Movements in the Minuet Fully Explained*, used written explanations of figures, along with simple floor movement patterns and illustrations of hand positions.

Global Modern

Ann Hutchinson Guest, in her 1998 book entitled, *Choreographics: A Comparison of Dance Notation Systems from the Fif-*

teenth Century to the Present, notes that most contemporary notational schemes attempt to record dancer movements in terms of body placement in space and time, some with the addition of projected body movement energy, power or force.

Strictly speaking, there are as many different kinds of dance notation as there are dance organizations, schools, instructors and competitors. Even so, it is my experience that most share a number of notational elements in common such as (1) some indication of the overall thematic composition structure (e.g. AB, ABA including rondos); (2) synchronized intergroup, intra-group, couple and solo movements; (3) canons; (4) floor patterns and individual movement pathways; (5) high and low points; (6) mirroring and shadowing positions; (7) unicentric movements of each dancer's body parts with reference to his or her body center; (8) polycentric movements involving the coordination of two or more body centers at the same time; (9) body tension and release; and (10) syncopation (see British Columbia Ministry of Education's *Dance 11 and 12-Performance Choreography Integrated Resource Package*, 1997, Appendix F - Glossary; and *Raper's Dance Dictionary for Social Dances*, both of which are good online resources for further definition of each of these elements). Today, however, two particular systems of dance notation have proven most useful in ballet and staged dance.

Labanotation

In his groundbreaking book, *Written Dance*, Rudolf von Laban envisioned dance as "movement choirs," which evolved into a detailed and innovative system of recording movement with which his name is linked today. Dr. Ann Hutchinson Guest, in her 1970 book entitled, *Labanotation: The System of Analyzing and Recording Movement*, championed Laban's work and made it readily available to the world. In essence, a central staff is used to represent the central body line with right and left columns indicating steps and leg, torso, arm and hand movements. The shapes of various surrounding block symbols indicate directions of movement. Black, dotted or striped shading indicate power (low, normal or high), and their length, the time duration of movements (and thereby also rhythm).

The Benesh System

Widely used by ballet production companies, Joan and Rudolf Benesh's dance notation system was first published in 1956 under the title, *An Introduction to Benesh Dance Notation*. Since then, the Benesh Institute has championed their work, and the Benesh dance notation system is being adapted for use in such diverse fields as medicine as a means of recording and studying movement behavior. The Benesh System uses a highly stylized, shorthand-like script, along with lines intersecting a cross-like representation of the body center at different points to represent body positions and together, produce a film-like movement recording.

Arthur Murray

Around 1920, a young and relatively inexperienced dance instructor named Murray Techman began offering inexpensive home dance instruction by distance correspondence course. The heart of his course was a series of simple time-movement foot diagrams supplemented in his now famous 1938 book, *How to Become a Good Dancer*, with dance, styling and figure descriptions as well as actual photographs. Unknowingly, Arthur Murray, as he was later called, resurrected the Greek system of dance notation and using it, began a popular revolution in dance notation, recording and using the recordings to teach popular American-style smooth and rhythm dances of the time. In essence, Murray popularized the first American ballroom and rhythm dance notation system. Its simplicity and practicality eventually caught the minds, bodies and hearts of over 20 million American dancers. In later versions of his work, like *Murray-Go-Round*, he attempted to further advance his notation, with some difficulty, to include amalgamations of figures and a few simple routines—in other words, dance choreography. Reading his publications carefully, it seems unlikely that Murray was actually aware of his resurrection of the Greek dance notation system though, in fact, this is what he accomplished. For example, all of his choreographic notations, like the Greeks', begin with movement of the left leg. Aware or not, Murray set the pattern for social, performance and competitive ballroom dance and later DanceSport notation and choreography as it is known today, and through that, also established a systematic way of recording somatic movements.

International Ballroom and Latin American Dance Notation

At about the same time that Arthur Murray began peddling dance correspondence courses and his dance notation system to the United States, British dance teachers, besieged by requests from students interested in learning dances introduced by American GIs in World War One, formed a ballroom branch of the Imperial Society of Teachers of Dance (ISTD). A committee of this new branch was assigned the task of reinterpreting and recording both American and European ballroom dances for European learners. ISTD dance notation used largely English-language-based descriptions with photographs. Being limited to three-figure amalgamations, these early descriptions often proved difficult to apply unless a student already largely knew the basic movements and figures involved. Nonetheless, this style of dance notation and choreography became firmly entrenched with the 1948 publication of *The Ballroom Technique*, and later with *The Revised Technique of Latin-American Dancing*.

My primary professional coach, Mr. Albert Franz, uses ISTD notation almost exclusively, which I have learned to use in a personalized shorthand form in my dance journals to record figures, amalgamations and routines that I want to remember. Note: ISTD recently announced that both books will be undergoing updating, though from what I can see, they will most likely continue this primarily English-language-based notation. In summary, International-style ballroom and Latin-American dancing, while danced by several magnitudes more dancers than the American style, relies heavily on a notational system based in the English language using a slowly but ever growing set of "standardized" abbreviations to describe: (1) the various positions of the body in relation to the feet, e.g. contrary body movement position (CBMP), promenade position (PP), and outside partner position (OP); (2) alignment of the feet in relation to the room; (3) turn, measured between the feet usually in eights, e.g. 1/8 turn to the right; (4) rise and fall (elevation and lowering that is developed through the feet, legs, torso, neck); (5) footwork [the part of the foot in contact with the floor, e.g. heel (H) or toe (T)]; (6) sway (inclination of the body away from the moving foot and towards the inside of a turn); (7) frame (poise and holds); and (8) syncopation (the deliberate disturbance of the timing pulse or accent, i.e. rhythm with slows (S) and quicks (Q) all in relation to (9) preceding and following figures, and with reference to (10) counterclockwise movement down a line of dance (LOD).

Contemporary DanceSport Notation and Choreography

Most DanceSport competitors, coaches and performance choreographers (e.g. those working for DanceSport hit TV shows) use some version of the ISTD ballroom and Latin-American notational system coupled with a dance floor figure procession diagram in which figures are given abbreviations like

NST for a natural spin turn and are described in the dancer's native language. My partner and I have used this method to record new figures and routines in our dance journals.

This system, archaic as it may seem, is fueled by an almost universal ban on videotaping at DanceSport performance and competition events. On the other hand, four new DanceSport notational system movements are beginning to appear. One is the result of the growing demand for video-based instruction. For example, a commercial outgrowth of USA Dance and DanceSport, "The Champions" series of instructional videotapes now includes complete, prescripted video practice routines and choreographed performance and competition routines. The second is based on recent attempts to digitize, integrate and computer-analyze silhouette-style graphic dance recordings. Another is following on the heels of computerized special effects cinematography. The last is grounded in an exponentially increasing consumer demand for virtual reality-based applications for entertainment, teaching and instruction.

Each of these "new" forms of notation are progressively richer and at the same time more technologically complex. Which, if any, will emerge dominant is at this time, anyone's guess. My inclination is that the latter, if developed to the point that one could actually experience an active routine in virtual reality *in one's own body*, would change contemporary dance notation and usher in a new era of richer, more robust somatic notation, significantly changing both dance and ultimately somatic therapy as we know them today.

One big hurdle for all DanceSport notation systems, however, is that there are usually six to eight or so couples on a competition dance floor, causing each couple to constantly modify prescripted movements or choreographed routines to avoid couple-couple interference (called "ungentlemanly conduct," a disqualifying criterion in DanceSport competition). It is this nature of DanceSport competition, like the Greek dance games, that empowers DanceSport in terms of being an evolving sport with persistent spectator expectation of seeing something new, unique or unusual. It is this, I believe, that will eventually elevate DanceSport, like Ice Dancing, into a different, yet more popular realm, much like classical ballet, (a popular spectator dance) and Olympic ice skating (a popular spectator sport).

Timing, Step, Rhythm, Footwork, Musical Expression and Progression

Unlike dance notations systems, (of which, as discussed above, there are currently many), musical notation is unitary, comprehensive, and easily comprehensible to most. For example, in musical notation, timing is defined as and denoted by, a time signature indicating the number of beats in a measure written above the type of note that receives one full beat. For example, the time signature 3/4 means three beats per measure and that a quarter note should last the duration of one complete beat. Tempo is the number of such measures per minute (or mpm) at which the music is played. Since dance is in many regards an extension of music, it would make sense that dance notation would at the least use, and at best simply add, bodily movement information to these musical term definitions. Unfortunately, this is not the case.

In dance terms, timing can mean musical timing of any pattern of accented and non-accented beats, dance tempo or even the length of time taken to transfer bodyweight onto the moving foot, e.g. slowly (S) or quickly (Q).

Similarly, musical rhythm commonly refers to the way in which sounds of varying length and accentuation are grouped into recurrent patterns, but, as stated in Louis C. Elson's 1905, *Elson's Music Dictionary*, and more recently in David Peñalosa's 2012 book, *The Clave Matrix: Afro-Cuban Rhythm: Its Principles and African Origins*, in dance notation, dance rhythm can include musical timing (the steady beat of the music) as well as temporary danceable claves, interpretable rhythms, repetitive or accented syncopated movements, or it can be used to summarize what is most catchy. For example, ISTD on occasion still uses the term "timing" to refer to any form of dance timing and "rhythm" to refer to musical timing. However, most contemporary DanceSport coaches I know use the term "timing" to refer to musical timing and "rhythm" to refer to dance rhythm, e.g. a combination of slow (S) and quick (Q) movements, like SQQ. Timing and tempo are closely allied to musical and dance rhythm—the word rhythm in Greek having a meaning more akin to "flow"— just as dance rhythm is closely allied to body movement.

Simple patterns, when repeated over and over, can have an

almost hypnotic effect. For this reason, dance rhythm has been called the heartbeat of music, the "pulse" that breathes life into both. As Schneider mentions in his 2002 online article entitled, "The Four Elements of Music - melody, harmony, rhythm and dynamics," it is usually this aspect of rhythm that people have in mind when they feel "connected" to the beat and state that the song, musicians and/or dancers have "got rhythm," meaning an electrifying quality, an aliveness connected to the beat and yet, at the same time, somehow transcending it.

Foot work, on the other hand, is generally accepted to mean placement of the foot (heel, ball, toe or whole foot) onto the floor in relation to the beat. Footwork can also include any resulting rise or fall of the foot, ankle, leg, trunk, neck or topline. ISTD and most DanceSport coaches I know use a set of alphanumeric footwork abbreviations. For example, "1HT" means to place the heel onto the floor during the first beat, followed immediately by weight transfer from heel to toe.

Musical expression is defined by dancers in different ways but for this work I will use my principle coach, Mr. Albert Franz's definition: The result of the effect of natural or contrary body movement position (CBMP), natural or contrary body movement (CBM), footwork, turn and sway. Mr. Franz has often told me that in his opinion, musical expression, sometimes called musicality, defines the essential character of a dance.

Progression is commonly referred to by both ISTD and DanceSport competitors in terms of three components: (1) direction of movement in relation to one's center of weight, (2) alignment of the body in relation to the dance floor and (3) counter-clockwise movement along the line of dance or LOD. With the addition of progression, musically expressed figures become a dance.

In its most basic form, DanceSport is denoted by recording each of the above elements. Based on these elements, DanceSport is generally divided into ten dance genres, namely: slow waltz, slow foxtrot, quickstep, tango and Viennese Waltz or fast waltz (the five ballroom dances), and rumba, cha-cha, samba, jive and paso doble (the five Latin-American dances).

CHOREOGRAPHY OF THE TEN COMPETITIVE DANCESPORT DANCES

Slow Waltz

The slow waltz is commonly considered the simplest DanceSport dance genre for most people to recognize and dance. The time signature is 3/4, indicating three beats to a measure or bar with a quarter note getting one beat and typically eight bars to a musical phrase. The USA DanceSport and National Dance Council of America's (NDSC) approved competition tempo is 28 to 30 measures per minute (mpm). Lillian Ray, in her 1933 book entitled, *Modern Ballroom Dancing*, notes that the first beat of every bar is characteristically accented, while the second and third are generally not.

The Ballroom Technique by the Imperial Society of Teachers of Dancing, originally published in 1994, designates waltz rhythm as all slows (notated "S"). Footwork generally involves stepping and transferring weight from heel to toe on the first beat (1HT), to the toe on the second beat (2T) and from toe to heel on the third (3TH) with late rise and fall, although rise can vary, sometimes substantially. Waltz, in general, is a dance of turn and sway emphasizes these elements. The slow waltz can be danced in a small area, the repetitive three steps being danced forward, backward, forward and backward in a "box," or progressively (either forward or backward) along the line-of-dance (LOD).

In a 1 April 1997 communiqué, professional dance instructor, Mr. Albert Franz, added that more experienced dancers will also be aware of, and record CBM and CBMP as well as heel turn and heel pull actions. Generally speaking, slow waltz has 6 named "compulsory" figures, 18 named advanced figures and 6 advanced variations commonly used in DanceSport competition as the basis of a waltz routine. These figures were originally listed in the 1994 publication of *The Ballroom Technique* and have been retained in subsequent revisions. Peter Buckman in his 1978 book *Let's Dance: Social, Ballroom and Folk Dancing* and Reynolds in *Ballroom Dancing: The Romance, Rhythm and Style* both agree that at its highest level slow waltz is a dance of enticing sensual pleasure with a veneer of aristocratic composure.

Slow Foxtrot

The slow foxtrot is perhaps the most danced and versatile of

DanceSport dance genres. The time signature is 4/4, indicating four beats to a measure with a quarter note getting one beat. There are 4 beats to a bar with no major accents. Instead, according to *The Ballroom Technique*, there are minor accents on the first and third beats of every bar and the first beat of every second and ninth bar which define the distinctive eight-bar slow foxtrot dance phrase. According to both the 2005 *NDCA Rules & Regulations* and the 2005 *USA DanceSport Rule Book*, slow foxtrot music is typically played at 28 to 30 mpm.

The slow foxtrot rhythm consists of countless amalgamated variations of the basic quick-quick-slow (QQS) rhythm where S foot placement and weight transfer take an entire 2 beats of music. Slow foxtrot, being danced in long phrases, allows for considerable variation in footwork as long as top line rise and fall correspond roughly to the phrases. Albert Franz, in a 1 April 1997 personal communiqué, said that it is actually a flat dance of illusory rise and fall created solely in the moving partner's ankles, making the overall effect reminiscent of Ice Dancing. In *The Ballroom Technique*, slow foxtrot is characterized as a gliding dance with not infrequent toe-toe steps and a strong sense of linear progression.

With experience, a slow foxtrot can be danced with a distinctive early ankle rise, strong CBM/CBMP, buttery smooth HT rises and TH falls, and pivots with a distinctive late sway giving the dance a dreamy, smooth, floating-on-ice-or-air quality. In general, the body turns less than in most of the other standard dances.

Slow foxtrot has 5 compulsory figures, 14 named advanced figures and 6 named advanced variations as listed and detailed in *The Ballroom Technique* (for more variations see Alex Moore's 1986 book, *Ballroom Dancing*). According to Peter Buckman and Albert Franz, at its highest level, it is a dance of balance, control and perfect complimentary partnership dancing, giving the illusion of dream-like Ice Dancing.

Quickstep

Stephenson describes quickstep as the British equivalent of the American foxtrot with Charleston variations. Quickstep is aptly named, with its 50 to 52 mpm tempo as specified in the 2005 *NDCA Rules & Regulations* and the 2005 USA Dance *DanceSport Rulebook*. Like slow foxtrot it uses 4/4 timing with four beats to a measure but has a distinct accent on the first and third beats of each measure. The 1994 ISTD publication, *The Ballroom Technique,* states that quickstep phrases can be quite variable but at advanced levels are typically four bars (16 beats) in duration.

Quickstep rhythm is highly syncopated and therefore quite variable in expression; the eight compulsory figures (many actually amalgamations of simple one and two-step movements) are variously danced in SQQ, SQQS, SQQSS and SQQSSS rhythm.

Generally speaking, quickstep footwork uses early but slow rise over three steps followed by quick but gentle lowering in one step, giving the feeling of rising up a roller coaster hill and then free-falling down. Reynolds states that as the second and third rising steps are taken on the toes, this can create an illusion of "body flight" that, when fully developed, is the competitive signature of this dance.

According to the 1994 reference, *The Ballroom Technique*, basic quickstep progresses with the man moving forward, backward, and laterally along LOD while facing diagonal to the nearest wall. Quickstep, while quite fast, still incorporates CBM, CBMP, HT, and TH actions along with skips, hops, runs and an endless variety of individualized kicks and flicks. In addition to its 8 named compulsory figures, quickstep, as specified in *The Ballroom Technique*, has 14 named advanced figures (many amalgamated) and 5 advanced named variations.

Moore and Reynolds agree that as the standard equivalent of the jive, at its highest level, quickstep is a dance of youthful joy for both dancers and viewers, especially when the illusion of body flight is clearly evident.

Tango

Reynolds reports that tango music, with its 2/4 time signature and all beats accented, is a dance of compelling, driven and demanding character. According to the NDCA *Rules and Regulations* and USA Dance *DanceSport Rulebook* of 2005, the official DanceSport tempo is 31 to 33 mpm. Its unusual QQS rhythm with half-beat Qs lends it an air of the unexpected.

The tango hold is low and close with the woman's position

shifted slightly further to the man's right than usual. In DanceSport, tango poise conveys the illusion of constant body tension. Footwork is based on continuously left-turning strong heel leads without rise or fall. Albert Franz says it has a "stalking character, not unlike that of a tiger slowly preparing to attack."

Moore adds that strong, early CBM and CBMP along with syncopated "links" (sudden body position shifts of the couple's feet, creating the illusion of a shift of the woman's body to the man's right) and pivots with leg and foot flicks, are used to further heighten viewer excitement. Albert Franz adds that while constantly curving, tango ultimately progresses along LOD with occasional short quick phrases danced against LOD, again, to produce the unexpected. According to *The Ballroom Technique*, DanceSport tango routines incorporate 7 basic compulsory figures, 13 named advanced figures, 7 advanced named variations, as well as, according to Reynolds, countless unnamed variations taken directly from the American and Argentine styles of this dance.

While the character of tango is said by Alex Moore to be "eccentric," Buckman, Moore and Reynolds all suggest that indications are that the genre is slowly recapturing its earliest sense of erotic enticement, sexual tension and quick changes in sexual feelings.

Viennese Waltz

An energetic yet graceful dance, Viennese or fast waltz music is so much faster than the slow waltz that the dance has only four compulsory figures: the Natural (right) Turn, the Reverse (left) Turn, and Forward and Backward Change figures, only two named advanced figures (the Natural and Reverse Fleckerl) and no named variations although a Contra Check is often used when changing from Reverse to Natural Fleckerl. According to Alex Moore, in championship competitions variations are neither expected nor necessarily appreciated. Like slow waltz, the time signature is 3/4, however, both Moore and Reynolds agree that the first beat is unvaryingly strongly accented, and it is challenging when danced at the fast 56 to 60 mpm competition tempo.

The hold is similar to the slow waltz and quickstep but the man's left arm is held slightly lower and wider. Classic Viennese Waltz has no foot rise; however, I am seeing increasing numbers of Italian DanceSport competitors using foot, ankle, body and even topline rise to create a secondary rhythm of slow, powerful, graceful rotation. While there is less body sway than in slow waltz, sway is more constant and is constantly changing. It is particularly interesting that the man and woman alternately dance the same figures in different directions, giving the dance the further illusion of perfect, yet ever-changing symmetry. Alex Moore, in his classic 1936 book, *Ballroom Dancing*, mentions the use of either toe or heel-toe pivots on the backward half of all turns to complete the illusion. Reynolds notes that Viennese Waltz's simplicity in terms of figures makes certain that the most minute technical details receive intense judge and viewer scrutiny.

Rumba

The rumba is a slow, sensual dance of passion and seduction. Mr. Albert Franz has often told me, "Provocative, Setsuko! Rumba is a dance of love! You must appear provocative!"

Rumba time signature is 4/4 with 4, 8 and 16 count phrases. Competition tempo is 28 to 31 mpm. According to Franz, emphasis is on the second of the four beats coincident with a split percussive "heart beat" creating a distinctive "one, two-two, three, four" beat. In the International style, there is a change of direction just after the split second beat. This, in association with movements taken using a released or lowered hip, creates a subtle "figure-of-eight" hip motion referred to as "Cuban motion" in the 1983 work, *The Revised Technique of Latin-American Dancing*.

Rumba rhythm is QQS. The basic hold for most Latin-American dances, including rumba, is closed face-to-face but not close, with the man placing his right hand on the woman's left shoulder blade, and the woman placing her left arm lightly above his curving arm on the top of his shoulder. *The Revised Technique of Latin-American Dancing* mentions common hold variations, including face-to-face promenade and side-to-side, either touching hands, finger tips or without contact.

Footwork is generally ball flat (BF) without rise or fall. Turns from CBMP are common, sway and CBM are not. "Weighted Connection" is used in order to create a separate QS body and topline rhythm—what Albert Franz in a 15 April 1998 communiqué described as a "gooey" or "rubber-bandy" look, slowly stretching open then suddenly and quickly closing.

While there are 12 compulsory figures, three basic movements underlie all: the basic Walk, Spiral and Hip-Twist. According to Mr. Franz in a 3 May 1998 communiqué, a DanceSport competitor who has good rhythm, Cuban motion and can execute these three basic movements generally commands the competition floor. There are five named advanced figures and seven named variations. Because of the variety of holds, there is considerable latitude for technique, especially with regard to torso, free arm and free-hand movement.

The 1983 version of *The Revised Technique of Latin-American Dancing* states that International-style Rumba, when well-danced, is not a place dance, rather it moves slowly along or against LOD.

Performance rumba portrays and sometimes even incorporates passion, desire, jealousy, rejection and pain or, as Reynolds on page 82 of his book, *Ballroom Dancing* so aptly sums it: "when a superbly trained and inspired couple dances the rumba, they act out a personal and complex love story - the man turns the woman toward him, she turns away only to turn back once more and give herself to him before he rejects her... "

Cha-Cha

Cha-cha is a happy, carefree, "cheeky" dance, considered by some to be the most exciting of the Latin-American group. Cha-

cha features the dancing couple involved in "flirtation."

The 2005 *NDCA Rules & Regulations* and 2005 USA Dance *DanceSport Rulebook* both list the time signature as 4/4 with 4, 8 and 16 count phrases danced at a 32 to 34 mpm competition tempo.

Stephenson and Iaccarino, in their 1980 book, *The Complete Book of Ballroom Dancing*, state that much of cha-cha's popularity is based on its metronome-like "ticking" beats. According to the 1983 version of *The Revised Technique of Latin-American Dancing*, the basic rhythm, SSQQS, is accomplished by the dancer with foot movements on the 2, 3, 4 and 1 beats; the corresponding time values are 1, 1 ,1/2, 1/2, and 1 respectively. In actual competition, according to Tony Meredith and Melanie Lapatin in a personal communiqué from 10 October 1996, syncopated rhythmic variations such as QQS and QQQQ are often included to lend "spice" to the dance.

Cha-cha hold, steps, figures and movements closely resemble those of rumba, although they are often executed with a "crisper," earlier transfer of weight. Cha-cha's signature feature is the Cha-Cha-Cha Chasse, a forward, backward or sideways movement complex of three steps in which the second step closes on the "and" count, followed on the third step by full transfer of weight. A popular attractive variation, which I like to use, involves a slight crossing action on the "and" when moving forward or backward. In this "Cha-Cha Cross" as it is sometimes called (patterned loosely on the popular Rumba Cross advanced competition variation), the toe of the back foot is placed near the heel of the front foot with the toe turned out. Otherwise, as documented in the 1983 publication, *The Revised Technique of Latin-American Dancing*, cha-cha footwork is BF without rise or fall.

Musical expression is quite similar, and often identical to rumba, as the cha-cha is historically a derivative of rumba. Albert Franz as well as Stephenson and Iaccarino state that cha-cha's 12 compulsory figures are based on the three basic rumba movements described earlier with the possible addition of the Cha-Cha-Cha Chasse. Cha-cha has six named advanced figures and seven named advanced variations, all of which I enjoy dancing.

At its highest level, cha-cha is often portrayed as a "tease" dance, with the woman presenting her body as the desired object, constantly inviting the man to pursue her.

Samba

Samba music is usually written in 2/4—alternatively 4/4—time; the tempo is listed at 50 mpm in the 2005 *NDCA Rules & Regulations* and 2005 USA Dance *DanceSport Rulebook*. It is danced in 4-count phrases with the aggregate musical emphasis on every fourth count. Mr. Franz, in a 24 April 1998 instruction, advised that this unusual accenting should be further enhanced by a brief whole-body stop motion. Mr. Franz, Reynolds and the 1983 version of *The Revised Technique of Latin-American Dancing* all agree that samba is a rhythmic delight with seven intrinsic rhythms in 2, 4, 6, 8, 10, 12, 14 and 16 count musical phrases, giving it the widest range of interpretive possibilities of any DanceSport dance. The basic rhythm is (1) SS; there is, however, (2) an alternative basic bounce in SaS (slow-ah-slow) rhythm. The other rhythms include (3) SQQ, (4) QQS, (5) SSQQS (a cha-cha rhythm), (6) QQQQ (Corta Jaca rhythm) and (7) SaSaSaS (slow-ah-slow-ah-slow-ah-slow, called Volta rhythm).

Samba is danced BF. Turning, swing and sway are remarkably similar to slow waltz. Samba, like cha-cha, has a constant, metronome-like tick expressed in the dance by a distinctive, quick pelvic tilt in the half-beat. While technically a closed hold dance, even basic compulsory figures are often danced traveling, open or side-by-side in a manner that requires amalgamated change steps making samba challenging and intriguing even for advanced competitors. Unlike most Latin-American dances, samba progresses along LOD.

Nine basic compulsory figures, five advanced named figures and nine advanced named variations are listed in the 1983 version of *The Revised Technique of Latin-American Dancing*.

At its highest level, samba appears as an intense, electrifying dance of wild physical and often sexual abandon; in fact, it is the result of a highly energetic but disciplined combination of five segmented body movements performed in seven seamlessly interwoven, syncopated rhythms.

Jive

In DanceSport, jive is traditionally last in a "Ten Dance"

competition, requiring competitors to always reserve some stamina for what many consider the most physically demanding DanceSport dance. According to The 2005 *NDCA Rules & Regulations* and 2005 USA Dance *DanceSport Rulebook*, jive is the only truly North American Latin-American dance (the rest are Caribbean and/or Spanish) and is closely related to American swing, boogie-woogie, jitterbug, bebop and rock 'n' roll with elements from twist, disco and hustle. Jive has a 4/4 time signature and is danced at 44 mpm (American-style East Coast swing is 34 to 36) with accent on the first and third beats of each measure in three-bar phrases.

Reynolds, as well as Alan and Anik Doucet in a personal communiqué on 29 September 1997, and Albert Franz in a personal communiqué on 17 April 1998 described jive rhythm as SSQQ but it can be danced in single, double and triple-time. Jive is danced BF. It has a characteristic quick body rise created by straightening the bent knees. This action is hard for many, including myself, to master. Danced in triple-time, jive has a distinctive syncopated chasse (side, close, side) as part of its basic step and is followed by a back rock with Cuban motion. Triple-time rhythm is often denoted aQaQ, where "a" is pronounced "ah," and represents collecting the body onto center, then placing weight into a flexing knee and, on the "Q," the quick straightening of the knee with body rise to the point that the body is actually off the ground. This, the most energetic style of jive, lends itself to fast foot kicks and flicks danced "on the rise," an audience hallmark of jive.

In *The Revised Technique of Latin-American Dancing*, jive is a lively, rotating, in-place dance in which the partners dance toward each other around a common center. To this, Franz and Reynolds add that, strictly speaking, jive has both CBMP and strong CBM, the latter consisting of a small torso and upper body turn in the opposite direction of the intended turn to garner pre-turn body tension and give speed and precision to turns, with the head following late. Rocks and spins accomplished with connection are part of the expected character of the dance, according to *The Revised Technique of Latin-American Dancing* and Reynolds.

Jive has nine basic compulsory figures, five advanced named figures and five advanced named variations. Given my early training in American swing, a movement I particularly enjoy is swiveling.

Reynolds praises jive, when danced at its highest level, as the epitome of fast, youthful exuberance.

Paso Doble

There has always been some confusion as to what exactly is being portrayed in paso doble. Reynolds explains that paso doble dancers present a matador and bull, but, in fact, in DanceSport, they depict the *torero* and his cape. In an actual bullfight, the *torero* weakens the bull by using his cape to entice it to participate in well-defined, particularly tiring movements; a matador's role is, quite simply, to kill the weakened bull.

The music used is that of the *paseillo*, the procession of the *toreros* into the bull ring, paso doble meaning "two step" in Spanish, Reynolds relates.

In DanceSport, paso doble is a dance of posture, the man dancing with the chest held high, the shoulders positioned wide and down, the head inclined forward. Body weight is kept well forward. Foot work is mainly BF, although many figures require the dancer to begin with a distinct heel lead followed by a pronounced body weight shift. While ostensibly without rise or fall, Albert Franz taught me the use of a slowly "unfolding" coordinated foot-ankle-knee-torso-neck rise to lend the dance a greater sense of drama. While the dance is popular throughout Spain, it is not easy to find paso doble music in strict 2/4 time at 60 to 62 mpm. I know. I've been to Spain in search of music to dance paso doble. The best music lends itself to four-count musical phrasing with every fourth beat emphasized as prescribed in the 2005 USA Dance *DanceSport Rulebook*.

Normally, one step is danced to each beat making the basic rhythm SS; however, both foot and body movements are often highly syncopated to increase the drama of the dance. Paso doble, emphasizing as it does the theatrical nature of dance, is commonly the last of the five Latin-American dances to be studied and learned. It is a quixotic dance in which the man, instead of the woman, strikes the dramatic poses using movements, lines, extensions and body-shaping to express the essence of this dance. The 1983 *The Revised Technique of Latin-American Dancing* states that CBMP, CBM and sway are often used to the extreme.

Varying patterns of steps and delayed heel-drops, coupled with complex, sinuous hand and finger movements borrowed from flamenco are on occasion, added to performances to refocus attention onto the female partner. They are, however, generally discouraged in competition, according to Franz.

The *Revised Technique of Latin-American Dancing*, released in 1983, states that paso doble is the only Latin-American dance which utilizes close, closed hold. It has ten basic compulsory figures, five advanced named figures and ten advanced named variations.

The reader might wonder at this point, why all the attention to the social dance and the details of choreography in the DanceSport versions of these dances? Restated, what does this have to do with somatic therapy? When I began my dancing career, I wasn't thinking about somatic therapy. At that time what I was searching for was key bodily movements and rhythms of life that made for perfect dance. Dance is after all, about movement and rhythm, and these seem to me linked to the very essence of what it means to be alive. It was later, after considering Dance Movement Therapy as a possible vocation, that I began to think of dance in broader terms, specifically, what my dance experience might reveal about my later vocational goal, the more elusive somatic therapy.

In fact, all the social partner and DanceSport dances I've mentioned so far actually do share a few rhythmic characteristics in common: First, they are all based on normal walking movements. Second, they each involve whole body expression through whole body movement. Third, they involve balance and posture. Fourth, they all present movement through time and space, in effect, active rather than passive movement.

At the same time, they represent basic classes of body movement. For example, the ballroom dances, namely waltz, foxtrot, tango, quickstep and Viennese Waltz involve not just individual movement but also partnership movement and balance ("two moving as one") as well as socialization, while the Latin dances, namely rumba, cha-cha, samba, jive and paso doble involve not just individual bodily movement but movement of energy from one partner to the other and back (the "gooey" connection), enlisting every muscle to express feeling, and using lead and follow.

Setsuko Tsuchiya

Chapter 3
Olympic DanceSport

I believe that it is time for DanceSport to become an Olympic event and continue to wait patiently for it to happen. While there is certainly a strong social aspect to partner dance, it can also be a performing art requiring and displaying a high level of individual athletic and technical skill. However, it is different from most other performing arts in that it is more primal. Not everyone draws, paints, sculpts, sings or plays an instrument, but everyone moves their body. World Professional Dance semifinalist and seven time North American Ten Dance Champion Mr. Albert Franz has repeatedly stated, "Dance is about musical expression—rhythmical movement through time and space." While social and keen amateur ballroom and Latin dancing is almost universal, its epitome can be expected in world Olympic competition.

While social activities bind people together, time and distance tend to separate. Each nation and era has its own dances and styles of expression, at least until just recently. Reynolds reminds us that social dance events have quite suddenly been transformed into unique social and national dance performances, to world dance, DanceSport and now one-world DanceSport.

In England in 1924, the Ballroom Branch of ISTD was founded to bring together the world's most popular social dances, codify, elaborate and perfect them into what is now known as the International-style of ballroom dance. Reynolds relates that very soon afterwards, society members began visiting Spain, Brazil, Haiti, Cuba and the nightclubs of Harlem in the USA to identify and organize the Latin-American dances. Social dancers responded by asking for lessons in these standardized dances so they could dance them with others anywhere in the world, ergo, world dance. For example, in April 1993, I met my future husband at a YMCA dance in Berkeley, California. We both enjoyed dancing, so we took social dance lessons together once a week. Two years later, when we moved to Hawaii, we were astounded that we could dance with people there as well as visiting dancers from throughout Europe, Asia and the Pacific.

Most dancers are social dancers and there are a surprising number of social dancers in the world. For example, when asked, Mr. Roger Izumigawa, at that time the Regional Representative to USA Dance, estimated there to be about 12,000 social dancers in 15 social dance clubs in Honolulu alone. Some social dancers study the standardized figures (syllabi) with or without professional instruction, while keen amateurs, often called novices, learn sufficiently about dancing to be able to move both comfortably and unobtrusively, paying special attention to their hold, poise and balance. Moore says that as these are mastered, keen amateurs usually turn their attention to rise and fall, turn, swing and sway. Daniel S. Janik, my competition partner, estimates that in Hawaii there are perhaps 120 keen amateurs—roughly one for about every 100 social dancers.

Keen amateurs with professional coaching and practice can become performance or competitive dancers, dancing for both personal and public pleasure; however, amateur performance and competition is often still seen by the public as social dance, something for old people.

Most competitive dancers in the USA in fact, compete "pro-am;" that is, they are judged "solo" against the syllabi (the professional they dance with is purportedly not judged). For example, a Japanese friend who lives in Hawaii had been taking dance lessons from a professional twice a week for the past four years because she didn't have a dance partner. When she competed in the Hawaii Star Ball, she entered the "Pro-Am" competition. At the same time, amateur-amateur couples were dancing, competing, and being judged, each couple against the other in skill/age "groups." By my estimate, there are, currently in Hawaii, about 20 registered amateur-amateur competing couples, approximately one couple for every 50 keen amateurs, representing less than one percent of social dancers. Besides keen amateur skills, amateur-amateur competitors concern themselves with ISTD's syllabi figures, including frame, top line, CBM, CBMP, figure precedes and follows, hip movement and student, associate, standard levels of figures and their basic variations as specified in the society's *The Ballroom Technique* and *The Revised Technique of*

Latin-American Dancing. For example, at the annual Hawaii Star Ball, amateur-amateur couples can compete against each other in ten dances in up to seven age categories at the Junior, Novice, Pre-Championship and Championship levels. To prove they are amateurs and not professionals, American amateur-amateur competitors must register with USA Dance.

EVOLVING DANCESPORT

Peter Pover, former president of USA Dance, relates that DanceSport is any and all forms of athletic dance, commonly referred to as ballroom or Latin-American dance in the USA that come out of social dancing but require specialized technical knowledge, discipline and superior muscle development. In 1989, DanceSport was first recognized as an international athletic sport.

As explained in the USA Dance *DanceSport Rulebook*, DanceSport is organized into amateur and professional divisions. In the USA, USA Dance is the officially recognized certifying body for amateur competitors—called USA DanceSport Athletes—while the National Dance Council of America (NDCA) is the primary certifying body for professional competitors—called Professionals.

Initially, USA Dance and NDCA fought to become the singular organization to certify both USA amateurs and professionals competing in national and international competitions. However, in 1957, the International DanceSport Federation (IDSF) was formed and immediately began organizing member associations at the national level throughout the world, in the process recognizing USA Dance as the sole certifying body for amateur competitions within the USA (see "DanceSport Steps into a New Future with IMG"). USA Dance, in return, created the United States Dance Sport Council (USDSC), establishing USA DanceSport and issuing the first official USA Dance *DanceSport Rulebook*. Under the rules of the USDSC and IDSF, a "Recognized Competition" is now a competition that has received the official sanction of a member organization of the IDSF and/or World Dance and Dance Sport Council (WD&DSC, the officially-recognized international sports federation for professionals, now known as the World Dance Council or WDC).

USA Dance still officially "sanctions" all amateur chapter, regional and national championships as well as other DanceSport competitions. It also acknowledges NDCA Recognized Competitions, though the acknowledgement has not always been mutual.

With the World Olympics once again reconsidering DanceSport as a World Olympic event, the struggle to control amateur *and* professional DanceSport is about to reach a crescendo. Olympic contestants by definition must be amateurs. However, throughout the rest of the world, the distinction between amateur and professional athletes continues to blur. In a 1 January 2017 message to all USA Dance DanceSport Athletes, USA Dance President Glenn G. Weiss announced, "For the first time ever the leadership will include professional dancers that make their living teaching and judging dance…USA Dance is no longer just an amateur organization. We are a dance organization that is in competition with other dance organizations. Soon we will also have a professional competitive division."

Olympic Ice Dancing

Professional DanceSport continues organizing and evolving, and so does amateur DanceSport, the highest level of amateur DanceSport being the World Olympics. In terms of World Olympics, DanceSport is most analogous to Ice Dance, which, while not an original Greek Olympic event for obvious reasons, has been an established Winter Olympic event since 1976. According to Rodrigues, ice dancers use all the basic elements of figure skating—use of edges, stroking, speed, smooth turns—as well as the principles of good dancing—posture, balance, partnering skill and fluid motion—to create a fully choreographed routine conveying overall artistic beauty that at the same time captures the essence of a particular dance. This is not an accident. DanceSport teachers taught Olympic ice skaters how to "dance on ice" and as such, were at least partly responsible for creating Ice Dance. Ice Dance is one of the most watched Olympic events because, as Reynolds points out, it "draws attention to dancing's superb role model of compromise, cooperation, and mutual [partner] respect."

DanceSport athletes, like Olympic ice dancers, must develop their muscles, usually under the guidance of a specially trained athletic coach. Ice dancers perform memorized groups of required figures according to syllabi, while interpreting the music, following the timing and expressing themselves musically. Most importantly, both DanceSport and Olympic Ice Dance (in its most popular and watched form) involve male and female athletes working together as one. Rodrigues specifically points out that most other Olympic sports are individual events and aren't this gender-equitable. Finally, the USA Dance *DanceSport Rulebook* reminds everyone that modern DanceSport competitive events are scored using the Skating System of judging.

DanceSport is however, different from Olympic Ice Dance in several important ways. First, DanceSport is safer. DanceSport is performed on a floating (cushioned) wood floor with soft, stable shoes with suede soles. Ice skating is performed on ice, a hard, often unforgiving surface, with skates with narrow, sharp blades. Also, DanceSport athletes are required to always keep one foot on the ground—lifts aren't permitted like they are in Ice Dance. Lifts and jumps are actions that make Ice Dance an outstanding spectator sport. Amateur DanceSport athletes, however, make up for this by incorporating more kinds and variations of figures on a floating floor than ice dancers can do on ice. Rodrigues, for example, notes that good Latin-American dancing always highlights Cuban hip motion, something difficult to portray on ice.

In addition, DanceSport costumes can be more elaborate and interesting, thereby appealing to more people, as they include both formal (standard) and highly provocative (Latin-American) costumes. For safety reasons, ice dancers' costumes must be simpler than ballroom dancers' costumes. For example, ice dancers cannot wear decorations on their arms. Similarly, while DanceSport costumes can use flashy rhinestones to catch the lights and attention of viewers, ice dancers can only use bright or shiny materials, again for safety reasons, conveys Reynolds. I also think that DanceSport is easier than Ice Dance for the audience to empathically "feel" and understand. DanceSport has two style categories (Ballroom and Latin-American) familiar to everyone who has danced, which includes the millions of people who social dance. Ice Dance, relates Human Kinetics, in the 2009 book, *The Sports Rules Book* (third edition), has three highly-technical categories (compulsory, original and free dance) that, according to Gerri Waibert in a 2002 editorial entitled "On Ice Judging Controversies and Conspiracies" in the January/February edition of *Blades on Ice* magazine, are hard for most people, including social skaters, to understand.

Olympic DanceSport

Rodrigues says that thirty years before DanceSport was conceived, Norman Martin, one of the founders of USABDA, now USA Dance, was already suggesting to the International Olympic Committee (IOC) that ballroom dance be recognized as a world Olympic event. In 1996, the Canadian Amateur Dancers Association (CADA) established the CADA Olympic Committee and began publicizing the idea. This began an explosion in public interest in performance and competitive dance that continues to the present. According to Plover, at IDSF's request, the IOC in 1997 recognized IDSF as the official international representative of DanceSport. In the USA, states began including "ballroom dancing" as an amateur competitive sport at the state level in pre-Olympic games—for example, the Aloha State Games in Hawaii, in which my partner and I competed. The ballroom dance competitions in the Aloha State games, the largest and most popular multi-sport competition in Hawaii, were hosted locally by USA Dance Honolulu on June 13th, 1998. Izumigawa in the November/December 1998 edition of Amateur Dancers related that ballroom dancing as a pre-Olympic competitive event was a success in his article "Aloha State Games a Success." Because of increasing public interest, IOC agreed to test the feasibility of DanceSport as a World Olympic event by scheduling an all-amateur DanceSport Exhibition in the 2000 Olympics Closing Ceremony. Don Herbison-Evans and his partner, Anna Piper, were two of the 1,000 dancers in the eight-minute "Love is in the Air" segment that aired before billions of Olympic viewers. "The energy exchange between us," states Herbison-Evans in his article "Eight Great Minutes" in the January/February 2002 edition of *Dancing USA*, "them [the Olympic athletes], the volunteers alongside them, and the audience at our backs, made a crescendo of emotion that turned the eight minutes into a triangle of dream, fantasy, and reality."

As K. C. Patrick reported in his February 2002 article in *Dance Magazine* entitled "Orphans and Olympians," because of the success of the exhibition, IOC showcased DanceSport again in the 2002 Olympic Arts Festival held continuously during the 2002 Olympic and Paralympic Winter Games. From February through March 17, the world witnessed some of the finest professional and amateur dancers from dance companies like Alvin Alley American Dance Theater, American Folk Ballet, AXIS Dance Company, Children's Dance Theatre, Savion Glover, Limon Dance Company, Pilobolus Dance Theatre, Repertory Dance Theatre, Ririe-Woodbury Dance Company and exhibitions of the Navajo Nation that mixed dance, athletics and gymnastics. DanceSport was designated as a World Game at the request of IOC because there reportedly wasn't room for any new Olympic events at least until 2008. The World Games (versus the Olympic Games) are held to honor all sports that have received full recognition by IOC and that are still awaiting a slot in an Olympic program; DanceSport had finally become elevated to such a sport. As a result, the sixth World Games, held on August 25 and 26, 2001, in Akita, Japan, included 48 couples competing in Standard and Latin-American DanceSport competition, representing 28 of the 73 countries participating in the world Olympics.

Now it's a waiting game. In the meantime, as Plover points out, the IDSF has entered a long-term joint venture agreement with Mark McCormack's International Management Group (IMG). IMG, IDSF's official commercial representative empowered to promote and handle all television, sponsorship and marketing rights, will produce eight major DanceSport competition events for airing throughout the world. On July 25, 1998, the first event was screened by the United States' National Broadcasting Company. At the screening, sport journalists were officially introduced to DanceSport and began to write and talk about it in major sports magazines and on the air; as a result, it was scheduled to be covered as a sport by the popular but conservative magazine, *Sports Illustrated*. Attention began turning to such athletic body characteristics as breathing, balance, posture, sensation, feeling, muscle strength and tone, active and passive range of motion, and motivation, all on an international scale. What can be expected to result is a new understanding of how to help athletes and thereby all people to more fully actualize their highest level of bodily function, similar in nature to Maslow's Hierarchy of Needs and athletic coach John Wooden's Pyramid of Success, in the process further defining the highest level of dance, DanceSport and thereby somatic therapy.

THE FUTURE

Khor Su Min, a new-age international sports reporter for *The New Paper*, in an August 1997 article entitled "Olympic Dreams Spurs Couple," reported online on the Singapore government's website NewspaperSG, "Ballroom dancing has got the green light to be included as a sporting event at the Olympics. But it's more than a sport..."

Reynolds adds in his book *Ballroom Dancing: The Romance, Rhythm and Style* on page 152: "For better or worse, North American mass media is on the verge of discovering

DanceSport and capturing its action, color, drama, sensuality and glamour for presentation to a wide audience...DanceSport cuts across ethnic and cultural lines like virtually no other competitive activity."

Reynolds continues that in recent years, ballroom dancing has been expanding steadily as both a performance and competitive sport, almost subversively, until it stands poised for an explosion of coverage by mass media. We are drawn to ballroom dancing, performed at the zenith of ardor and skill because the participants move our souls. Yes, we are dancers all, and this is what makes social dance, keen amateur dance, and amateur performance and competition DanceSport universally applicable. It is this universal applicability that suggests to me that dance must play a role, most likely a major one, in somatic therapy.

If dancing in its social form is a natural amusement, providing enjoyment and exercise, it has slowly begun changing from a social pastime to a world-class, competitive sport. It is this latter form, through research and experimentation, that many of the qualitative characteristics of dance are being transformed into quantitative elements and the relative contributions of each element are being applied to overall body function, performance, training, endurance and reserve. These are all key aspects of body protection and preservation, contributing to a person's health, recovery and actualization. So where does amateur competitive DanceSport stand today? The World DanceSport Federation posted a press release on 29 June 2015 on their website, confirming that DanceSport will not appear in the 2020 Tokyo Olympics.

However, it will appear on the short list of contested sports and, having generated more revenue than any other contested sport in the 2009 and 2013 World Games, DanceSport as a future World Olympic event appears more than promising.

Aside from the social appeal, glamour and flash, what is it about dance that then makes it important to somatic therapy? I took up social dance, competitive and performance dance, then DanceSport as a pastime and whole body exercise, a way to maximize my health, retain my passion for life and prevent illness and aging. In the process, however, I came to realize that dance, especially couple dance, has some particularly interesting attributes:

It maintains mental acuity and memory.

It promotes awareness of internal rhythm.

It encourages good posture and deep breathing.

It includes human-to-human touch.

It supports social connectivity.

It provides a creative outlet.

It creates a pathway for the expression of joy.

All of these particular attributes suggested to me that dance might indeed prove to be an ideal way to prevent physical illness and disease, promote natural healing and prevent many of the effects of aging. In addition, over the years, I have come to believe that in doing so, it might actually serve as a way to maintain mental health, to attain innate needs, wants and desires for self-actualization and possibly serve as a complementary or even alternative approach to healing both physical and mental disorders.

If so, it would, in addition, provide one particularly interesting characteristic: It would be language-free. That is, it would be an approach to physical, mental, social and spiritual health that is body-based, rather than dependent on spoken communication. This might provide a way for people of different cultures, races, ages, genders and languages, to "communicate" directly with their bodies and even body-to-body rather than through an interpreter, translator, psychologist or counselor.

Chapter 4
I Want to be a Dance Movement Therapist

I initially regarded dance as an avocation, but as I progressed in my dancing, I began exploring ways to share with others what seemed to me the powerfully positive attributes of dance. It was during this period that I ran across an article in *Dance View*, a periodical Japanese dance magazine, about a new occupation called "dance movement therapy." In 1998, I enrolled in an American college (though English is my second language—Japanese is my "mother tongue"). While an Associate of Arts in Liberal Arts and Studies student at Thomas Edison State College (now Thomas Edison State University or TESU), I took a class entitled "Living in the Information Age," a part of which involved exploring career opportunities using the US Bureau of Labor Statistics' *Occupational Outlook Handbook*. I focused my initial search on career opportunities in dance, looking also for dance movement therapy; however, the former resulted mainly in opportunities to teach dance or become a recreational dance instructor and the latter was not listed at all. This piqued my interest. The nearest category match, "Dancers and Choreographers," was devoted almost entirely to performing arts and/or dance instruction, neither of which addressed my greater interest in sharing what I saw as the special attributes of dance. Numerous searches later, I came across references to "recreational therapist," "physical therapist," "athletic trainer," "counselor," and just "therapist" in general. However, none seemed to fit. I wasn't interested in being an "athletic trainer," or a counselor or therapist. Finally, I did a Google search on "How to become a Dance Therapist" and found out that the American Dance Therapy Association (ADTA) "sets and monitors standards for the master's level programs." According to ADTA, if one wants to become a Dance Movement Therapist he or she needs a Master's degree, preferably in Dance Movement Therapy.

For the moment, I chose Dance Movement Therapist as my occupational goal. TESU, however, did not offer a specific course of study in dance movement therapy that would address the academic requirements mentioned by the ADTA, so I had to take additional courses from Brigham Young University, Weber State University, former Heald College, Upper Iowa University and Argosy University. My goal was to study at the best university for each topic course, with professors known for their expertise in the various aspects of dance movement therapy.

During my studies, I asked my spouse, a physician, about how to best proceed, and he asked one of his colleagues, a physiatrist. They replied that actually, Dance Movement Therapy as a profession was still rather new. They recommended I study more about the body and, in the process, obtain a license to practice massage therapy. After completing my Associate of Arts Degree, I continued studying towards a Bachelor of Arts in Liberal Arts in Dance at TESU, and, during this time, I also enrolled at the Hawaii College of Health Sciences. I studied hard and qualified to take the state massage therapist examination in Hawaii. I passed the examination in 2004 and began applying all I'd learned in private practice as a licensed massage therapist.

While working as a massage therapist, I continued my academic studies in dance and psychology. During this time, I began applying what I was learning in anatomy, physiology and kinesiology to both massage and dance. Being a dancer was especially helpful in making me more sensitive to individual muscle movement. In my practice of massage therapy, I initially focused on Swedish massage.

Per Henrik Ling is generally credited with having developed "Swedish massage," which had been practiced in one form or another since Hippocrates described the benefits of anatripsis (meaning "to rub up") around 450 BCE. Ling's system of massage was based on the positions and movements of Swedish gymnasts. It included passive, duplicated and active elements. Sandy Fritz in her classic textbook, *Mosby's Fundamentals of Therapeutic Massage*, described the main passive movements as stretching and range of motion performed on a client by a trained gymnast (called a "therapist"), duplicated movements as oppositional efforts by both parties, and active movements purely by the client. Dr. Johann Mezger, a Dutch physician in the late 1800s, provided a medical explanation of Ling's movements, adding *ef-*

feurage (large gliding strokes applied horizontally with light to moderate pressure), *petrissage* ("kneeding;" lifting, rolling and squeezing applied vertically), and *tapotement* ("percussion;" application of springy light to heavy blows to the body at a specified rate). More recently, Swedish massage is said to also include compression, vibration and friction, making up a full complement of soft tissue "manipulation."

After mastering Swedish massage, I let myself explore the range of massage "manipulation" more widely, and, being Japanese, acupressure. Sandy Fritz defines acupressure as a modified version of acupuncture, using pressure rather than needles to stimulate certain points along ancient Chinese and Indian meridians (channels) and AhShi ("ouch") points outside the meridians. Acupressure, sometimes called "trigger point massage" in the West, involves the release of points of local nerve, muscle and connective tissue tension, typically called "microspasms."

During the next couple years, I combined Swedish and Trigger Point massage with my knowledge of dance and began offering "sports massage" to social, keen, performance and competitive dancers. It was during this time that I realized that problems of posture, breathing, mental imaging and balance, especially in partner dance, were at the root of many of the problems being presented. In particular, mental imaging by the client of the tense or painful area, and its release and relaxed sensation, proved an especially effective adjunct to massage. Clients experiencing too much pain for direct or indirect manipulation seemed to especially benefit from this trio of mental imaging, repeated active release and awareness of the released sensation. To explore this further, I studied Reiki. Reiki uses near or light touch to initiate reflexive body energy responses. I found Reiki, though less effective, particularly intriguing.

I received my Bachelor of Arts Degree in Liberal Arts in Dance from TESU in 2010 and began making plans to attend an American university offering a Master's degree in Dance Movement Therapy. It was at this time, I became aware of the profound implications of a difference in emphasis between the "dance," "movement" and "therapy" in Dance Movement Therapy. What I discovered was that most American universities offering a Master's degree in Dance Movement Therapy emphasized psychological "talk therapy" over actual bodily movement and/or dance, the more somatic elements. Also, most, when utilizing dance or dance movements, typically applied individual, modern ("jazz") dance movements. None specifically emphasized the application of the attributes of dance that I thought made couple dance so ubiquitous and potentially therapeutic. If the answers weren't in contemporary schools of dance movement therapy, then I would have to delve deeper into its earliest historical roots before it became so focused on psychology.

Setsuko Tsuchiya

Chapter 5
Pythagoras and Eurythmy

Having become fascinated by dance, massage, dance movement therapy and all their therapeutic ramifications, I found myself asking why they have the positive affect that they do on people. That is, what, if anything, do they share in common that is "therapeutic?" My historical research has led me to believe the answer is related to the Pythagorean concept of eurythmy. I came upon this revelation when I was listening to a lecture by Dr. Daniel S. Janik, who was at the time an instructor of undergraduate studies at Argosy University Hawaii, teaching a Science 110 course entitled "The Rise of Modern Science." He said that Pythagoras was one of the first and perhaps greatest of the Greek philosophers, as well as the father of science, mathematics and, to my surprise, therapeutic music. Pythagoras never personally recorded his theories, but is attributed by others after him as having been the first to determine that the pitch of a musical note occurs in proportion to the length of a string that produces it, that intervals between harmonious sounds form simple numerical ratios, that all things emanate their own unique vibration and that the harmony of these vibrations ultimately determines the physical health and lives of individuals, planets, even the cosmos.

At the beginning of the 20th century, archeologists discovered many ancient Greek vases with depictions of dancing maenads. As these vases began to circulate in Europe, interest in Pythagorean beliefs resurfaced under the name eurythmy. Hans Fors, an eurythmist who taught at the Eurythmy School in Jaerna, Sweden, from 1979 to 1999, is cited in an internet article entitled "Repeating or Rejuvenating? The Beginnings of Eurythmy That Shape the Present," as saying that the word "eurythmy" in the ancient Greek tradition means a combination of rhythmic movement, music, speaking, line and color. While there is no direct evidence that Pythagoras ever used the word "eurythmy," he certainly seems to have invented the idea.

In 1918, Suzanne Perrottet started the first modern "school for eurythmy" in Zurich, Switzerland, and taught music, singing, rhythmic gymnastics and emotional forms of movement, including dance. While the idea of eurythmy was new to many modern Europeans, it seemed derived from ancient Pythagorean beliefs.

First, ancient Greeks, like Pythagoras, believed that natural, rhythmic body movement—that is, dancing and singing to music in artful surroundings—was the highest form of expression. According to Dr. Maurice Emmanuel, Professor of Dance at the Paris Conservatory, in his book titled *The Antique Greek Dance*, the ancient Greeks danced at births, weddings, celebrations and deaths. They even danced to commemorate battles; their "battle" dances were eventually called Pyrrhic dance. The special quality of ancient Greek dance was "a very keen sense of mimetic value, joined to perfect rhythm." Perfect rhythm—the Rhythm of the Spheres—was what Pythagoras thought made mathematics, music, people and the cosmos work. In fact, John N. Clayton in "The Dance of the Spheres," an internet article dated January/ February 1999, said, "Dancing to the music of the spheres was an activity that occupied much of the time of the ancient Pythagoreans."

Second, Pythagoras used music, and presumably dance, to heal. Dr. James J. Garber MD PhD in his book, *Harmony in Healing: The Theoretical Basis of Ancient and Medieval Medicine*, mentions that Pythagoras used movement and music to soothe both animals and people. He goes on to say that Pythagoras is considered by many to be the founder of music therapy. Recognizing the profound affect of music upon the senses and emotions, Pythagoras did not hesitate to influence both mind and body with what he is said to have termed "musical medicine." Modern Dance Movement Therapy (DMT) uses natural and unnatural body movements, many taken from ancient as well as modern individual, interpretive jazz and contemporary dance, to treat illnesses of the body and mind.

Third, eurythmy involves perfect proportion in movement, sound, color and design. According to Rudolf Steiner in his book, *A Lecture on Eurythmy*, the Greeks and Romans used the word "eurythmy" [ευ (eu: beauty), ρυθμός (rhythms: rhythm)] to represent perfect, harmonious visual proportions in design.

In short, while the idea of eurythmy was new to 20th century Europeans, it actually began centuries earlier with Pythagoras. Dr. Emmanuel, on page 304 of his book says, "With the Greeks the dance was an art much more highly regarded than with us. The philosophers attributed to it a moral influence; they said that 'the dance is, of all musical arts, the one that most influences the soul'."

Pythagoras was not only the father of science, mathematics and music but also, in my mind, the father of eurythmy. Two thousand five hundred years ago, he knew that dance was the highest expression of the body, mind and soul, incorporating it into the Pythagorean mysteries along with music and song. But his most important contribution, I think, is the introduction of the idea of rhythm as a method of healing, and that typically more than one rhythmic healing element needs to come together in perfect order to be most effective.

Margarete Kirchner-Bockholt, in her 2007 book entitled *Foundations of Curative Eurythmy*, states that eurythmy is an expression of each human leading a "rhythmic life." Frequently quoting Rudolf Steiner, she roughly divides rhythmic life into physical, mental and astral or spiritual rhythms. Within the physical rhythms she includes organ rhythms such as breathing (lungs), circulation (heart and vessels), digestion (upper and lower digestive system) and muscular exercise, including stepping, bending and stretching. To these I would add dancing, massage, and the female and male procreative rhythms, as well as individual mental rhythms, for example, wakefulness (attentiveness to the environment) and sleeping (inattentiveness to the environment). Kirchner-Bockholt states on page 94 of her book that the "characteristic of all rhythmical processes is that they do not go on forever, but turn rhythmically inwards upon themselves." Expanding on her statement, these life rhythms can be repetitively cyclical or spiral in nature, spiral rhythms being inward directed (consciousness), outward directed (expression), upward directed (renewal, gestational or nurturing) or downward directed (dissolution, aging and death).

Of these "rhythms," one that consistently appears central to both dancing and massage is breathing. The ancient Greeks held that the psyche—that which animates the body—is in fact the breath. It was Dr. Wilhelm Reich, a colleague of Dr. Sigmund Freud, who brought these various concepts together and, as I like to say, "freed the body from the tyranny of the mind" with his distinctly somatic theory of health based on energy entrapment and its release through movement.

Setsuko Tsuchiya

Chapter 6
Wilhelm Reich and Body Therapy

Michel Cattier, in his seminal work translated from French to English and published in 1971, *The Life & Work of Wilhelm Reich*, tells us that Wilhelm Reich, born 1897 and died 1957, was one of the most challenging and revolutionary thinkers of the twentieth century. He was a physician and Freudian psychoanalyst who eventually emigrated from Vienna to the United States.

In 1920, while attending medical school, he began working in Freud's second psychoanalytic outpatient clinic, the Vienna Ambulatorium, advancing quickly to the position of Assistant Director. A member of the "inner circle" of Freud's Vienna Psychoanalytic Society, he expressed a keen interest in character, ego defense and sexuality and wrote extensively on all three.

Reich spoke publicly against any form of institutionalized authority, emphasizing instead the need for each individual to achieve and maintain free flow of energy, including sexual energy.

While he and Freud initially shared Freud's theory, or at least very similar theories of psychoanalysis, they eventually came to see things quite differently. Freud felt that mental problems resulted in physical signs and symptoms, and stressed "talk" therapy and through it, release of body signs and symptoms. Reich, on the other hand, came to believe that mental problems resulted from trapped physical energy and through release of that energy, resolution of mental problems. In addition, he stressed prevention on a societal scale. According to Reich, character (muscular) "armor" was an observable physical property that clients, with help, could feel. Psychoanalysts could observe this trapped energy as muscular rigidity. "Character resistances," says Cattier on page 196, "are thus riveted in the inflexibility which affects certain selected groups of muscles." Cattier, on page 58, offers that Freud believed, "'civilization'…is built by abstract individuals who channel their sexual energy into their work," while Reich on the other hand, held that "only a minority of people are able to 'sublimate' their sexual needs, while others become neurotics whose work capacity diminishes."

As such, in 1927, Reich began organizing mental health centers where parents and youth could receive information on sexual physiology and contraception. As Cattier explains, his work with families and adolescents was slowly leading him to the conclusion that the common "cause" of adolescent sexual frustration was the nuclear family, a conclusion that quickly generated opposition.

Reich called directly upon his medical practice, research and knowledge, publishing profusely on both his unique approach to psychotherapy while attempting to identify its distinctive biophysical (today, neurobiological) foundations. His later experiments in "orgone energy" entrapment using an "orgone accumulator" brought him into conflict with the United States Food and Drug Administration, leading eventually to imprisonment and the destruction of many, if not most, of his works. Today, such destruction of books would seem inappropriate. It is likely that in addition to his refusal to stop producing and selling accumulators, his unsavory history with the Communist Party, his emphasis on sex and sex treatment as being at the root of neuroses, his fearlessness in touching his clients and his denigration of the family, all may have played a part in the court's unusually draconian decision. His remaining works are available from the Archives of the Orgone Institute in Rangeley, Maine.

John P. Conger expressed Reich's unique psychotherapeutic approach on page xvi in his 1994 book entitled, *The Body in Recovery - Somatic Psychotherapy and the Self,* where he says, "Our body faithfully records the traumatic events in contracted musculature and energetically withdrawn tissue."

Traumatic events, whether physical, sexual or psychic, not only result in persistent physical contractions of muscles, but also a "blockage of energy flow," that, if severe enough, can cause victims to split what should be a cohesive life into the disintegrated experience of different bodies such as the birth, infant, child, teen, young adult, adult, old and very old body. It is for example, this felt sense of splitting that leads to psychoses. Most trauma, however, does not necessarily result in sensory disintegration of the body, but rather results in energy blockage and muscle contraction, which in turn cause mental anguish.

On page xvii, Conger also says, "There have been two paths in body therapy. In the first path or 'character' as Reich called it, to unblock the body structure so that the body's healthy rhythms can awaken or reassert themselves. In the second path, supportive attention calls forth the hidden resources of healthy functioning to throw off the body's unnecessary encumbrances."

To repeat, Reich's approach was the polar opposite of Freud's. For Reich, body signs and symptoms were directly caused by the blockage of orgasmic life energy, which in turn caused mental stress and problems. Although he never proved the existence of "orgone" energy to the satisfaction of Freud, the members of the Vienna Psychoanalytic Society or the medical community at large, he was nonetheless a pioneer in attempting to provide a true neurobiological foundation for the primary use of somatic rather than "talk" treatment in the field of mental health. Furthermore, he emphasized prevention over treatment of mental problems through the application of individual and social interventions.

It is interesting to note that to be considered a psychoanalyst at that time, one had to first be psychoanalyzed by a member of the society. The idea was that this would allow a psychoanalyst to become aware of his or her own problems and thereby avoid transferring them to patients (transference). Freud psychoanalyzed himself, so it can be loosely said that all traditional Freudian psychoanalysts have been indirectly psychoanalyzed by Freud. In actuality, Reich was psychoanalyzed by Isadore Sadger, one of Freud's earlier followers who had a special interest in sexuality. Reich later psychoanalyzed Fritz Perls, the founder of Gestalt psychology and one of the contributors to humanistic and transpersonal counseling psychologies, which remain popular today.

According to Conger, Reich believed we are "emotionally present" until subjected to the repressive behavior of caretakers. In response, we produce a "false self" which Reich called "character." The first step to resolving the marshaled physical defenses of this new character is "contact." Contact, in Reichean terms meant more than just talking. It required visual and tactile contact, along with grounding, boundary identification and respect, "unrestricted breathing" and intent to remain in the present.

According to Reich, anxiety represented blocked libidinal energy, which is expressed directly in the body. For example, he regarded contraction of the diaphragm and breath-holding as early mechanisms used to suppress sensations resulting in anxiety and its necessary release. Reich, according to Conger, referred to these physical defense mechanisms as "body armor."

Conger relates that to treat this condition, Reich typically applied gentle pressure with his fingers between the center of the ribcage and the navel. This physical contact resulted in relaxation of abdominal muscles, allowing deeper diaphragmatic and pelvic breathing. Reich believed that such "uninhibited breathing" led directly to orgasmic release, which he regarded as a physical reflex. It was his goal to physically locate points of inhibitions to the orgasmic energy flow and reflex, and: (1) intensify involved muscular contraction; (2) have the client breathe into the intensified contraction; (3) and/or massage the area to assist in its deinhibition. These areas of inhibition, however, needed to be identified and released in a particular physical sequence to avoid repetition of trauma. In short, he worked with the upper body before attending to the principal common site of inhibition—the pelvis.

Conger further relates that Reich generally worked on seven successive "segments," beginning with eye contact and touch ("ocular segment"), followed by the oral segment, then cervical, thoracic, diaphragmatic, abdominal segments and finally the pelvic segment. He held it important to address these segments in association with deep breathing, with the client lying down. This could only be done physically, as the expressive biological language of the "core," meaning pelvic or orgasmic, was far beyond the reach of words. Addressing the core required not talk, but silence—a stillness of observation called "silent observation"—necessary for the client to marshal his or her natural life force resources in order to free himself or herself of the inhibitions. As these inhibitions were freed, the client would no longer need to cling to his or her mental anguish.

Reich said that orgone energy acts like a fluid. That is, it is constantly coursing throughout the body. When it becomes stuck somewhere, the person experiences physical and if left untreated, mental problems. Effective treatment of mental signs and symptoms therefore requires the "freeing" of these blockages, typically through the laying on of hands. Reich was noted to have experimented with massage on unclothed patients to dissolve muscular blockages, later referred to as "muscular armor." This went solidly against the belief among most psychoanalysts of not interacting physically with patients in order to protect against transference and counter-transference. This approach later led Reich to become marginalized within the psychoanalytic and later psychological communities.

His book, *The Function of the Orgasm*, published initially in 1927 and emphasizing the importance of natural or assisted orgasmic release, made him decidedly unpopular within the society. Reich's second analyst, Paul Federn, was said to have eventually come to regard Reich as a psychopath.

Reich later claimed that orgone was actually part of a greater "cosmic" energy—what some might regard as "God"—and this cosmic energy was behind the very life process, as well as things such as the color of the sky, gravity and the failure of most political revolutions. Inside living beings, Reich considered orgone a specially-adapted form of cosmic energy, namely orgasmic energy that needs regular release, and is equal or at least similar to Prana, Mana, Chi, Bio-Energy, Ki, Spiritual Vitality, ether and life force.

Reich came to conclude that not only mental illnesses, but many physical diseases, such as cancer, were caused by blockages of orgone in the body. This led him to develop specially designed "orgone accumulators" to collect orgone energy from the environment that could be used to focus and direct this energy to overcome blockages in individuals.

Wilhelm Reich may have been one of the first Western psychologists to associate Eastern ideas of medicine, involving energy and energy flow, with Western ideas of disease and mental illness. His later ideas may sound crazy, but Eastern medical practitioners and academicians have, for centuries, believed in and treated blockages of energy, some not unlike orgone, flowing along established pathways within the human body, often connecting the body with the world and cosmos. Western medicine conservatively calls these biological energy accumulators and pathways nervous tissue and nerves; Eastern medicine calls them chakras, meridians and channels. Interestingly, nerves, meridians and channels appear, in some instances, to share common physiological pathways within the body, while in other cases, none at all. I believe that body therapy is important for the treatment of ill and diseased patients, whether the illness or disease is physical or mental. As a medically-trained and licensed massage therapist, I can easily imagine my work involving some kind of life force or energy flow each time I do a massage.

While evidence for general, spiritual, sexual, life or cosmic energy remains elusive, at least in a Western scientific sense, people today receive "somatic" therapy in the form of acupuncture, acupressure, Reiki, Rolfing, Swedish deep tissue massage and Lomilomi, to mention only a few, all which claim to be based directly or indirectly on some form of energy and/or energy movement. More to the point, patients have reported experiencing health benefits, and more recently, evidence has begun to accumulate suggesting somatic therapies have reproducible affects on respiration, heart rate, blood pressure and attitude. This lends support to Reich's basic concept of a general life force and the importance of treating the body to treat the mind. The United States National Institutes of Health's National Center for Complementary and Alternative Medicine (NCCAM) includes on its website Reichian-style body therapies like tai chi, gi gong, healing touch, yoga, chiropractic and osteopathic manipulation, body-based relaxation techniques and body movement therapies such as Trager/Alexander/Feldenkais/Aston massage, Rolfing and Pilates as complementary and alternative medical treatments. To these, Sandy Fritz adds myofacial release, anma, Lomilomi, reflexology, Do-in, Jin Shin Do, Jin Shin Jyutsu, sports/medical/infant massage. To all of these I have to add Neotantric/navatantric massage because of its full circle return to Reich's fundamental principle of somatic sexual release. I believe that, as the idea that treating the body can also heal the mind becomes more contemporary, the biological bases of CAM therapies will be further elucidated.

The reader might ask at this point, how does eurythmia fit into Reich's concept of healing the body to heal the mind? To the best of my knowledge, Reich never mentioned eurythmia directly; however, he repeatedly mentioned and used both passive and active movement in his practice, specifically to unblock energy as he moved his clients through the seven successive segments. While he may have used it in conjunction with talk therapy, he repeatedly emphasized the importance of directly interacting with the body rather than with the unconscious or conscious mind. As a speaker of English as a second language, it struck me as particularly interesting and powerful that when using a Reichean approach, language differences no longer presented a barrier like they do with talk therapies. Furthermore, as a massage therapist and more importantly, a dancer, I became interested in furthering his concept of segmental movement to that of graduated, whole body, eurythmic movement as a more holistic form of body therapy.

Chapter 7
The Power of Dance

As previously mentioned, dancing can be a powerful method of non-verbal communication. Furthermore, while many argue that language is a form of communication only available to humans, dance interestingly is not. Most, if not all, animals dance! They might dance to impress potential mates or fend off attackers. As people (we are after all first animals, then humans), we can certainly use dance to accomplish these purposes. In fact, we often break into spontaneous dance to express our joy when having a good time. We can easily find ourselves dancing to catchy songs, even to ones that do not contain any lyrics. Music adds rhythm of sound to body rhythm through variations in the length and accentuation of sounds. With such diversity of expression—consider, for example, the Nutcracker ballet, a game of "charades" or a pantomime (when done by Marcel Marceau, clearly a form of dance)—one can communicate even the most complex of ideas and emotions through dance.

People, young or old, move their body. It's just part of being a human animal. My first competition DanceSport instructor and coach, Mr. Albert Franz, said, "Dancing is movement through time and space. In fact I have expressed feelings of happiness and sadness through dancing using...body movement."

Dancing is said to have co-originated alongside culture and society, being associated with weddings, celebrations and funerals; people attending these events were thought to dance their happiness or sadness. At such events, people of different countries often dance together and in the process come to understand each other's feelings and culture better. Often they add color in the form of costumes, and pass the increasingly elaborate tradition from generation to generation.

Dancing was thought to be present before, and even transcend spoken language. For example, not far from my house, the Mo'ili'ili' Community Center holds an annual Summer Festival that includes bon dancing. Originating in Japan, people of any ethnic and cultural background can join in and enjoy copying and dancing with Japanese music without ever understanding the Japanese meaning of the song. Participants enjoy the individually felt sensation of seasonal festival dance.

In summary, dancing—moving one's body through time and space—is innate to the human as well as the human animal and represents a distinctive form of non-verbal communication—using body movement to convey feelings with rhythm, timing and footwork. No one wants to forget the dances of their own society and culture. Dancing, in this sense, is life itself, or stated in a Reichean manner, the act of living through the movement of life-giving energy.

It was in the 1950s that dance first began to be recognized not only as a form of social interaction, artistic expression and competition, but also a distinctive form of body communication that provided insight into human thoughts and behavior. This common idea developed differently on the West and East Coasts of the United States of America, the former under the influence of Mary Starks Whitehouse ("Authentic Movement") and the latter under the influence of Marian Chace (Dance Movement Therapy).

Mary Starks Whitehouse in a 1958 lecture entitled "The Tao of Body" quoted on page 241 of Don Hanlon Johnson's 1995 book, *Bone, Breath, & Gesture - Practices of Embodiment*, is said to have emphasized that "animals…have their being in movement, exist by virtue of it, [and] show forth their nature through it." She identifies breathing, circulation, digestion and reproduction as key parts of this movement. On page 242, she is said to have specifically stated: "Two things about physical movement are striking: One is that movement is non-verbal and yet it communicates" and so "the body does not, I would almost say cannot, lie." On the same page, she explains her latter statement to mean that whatever a physical body is doing can't be hidden by "words, by clothes, least of all by wishes." In this sense, physical movement is one of the most fundamental forms of expression. That includes psychological expression. In short, "just as the body changes in the course of working with the psyche, so *the psyche changes in the course of working with the body*" (the italics are mine), leading her to the conclusion that the "core of movement experience is the [felt] sensation of moving and being moved." In summary, movement, in her opinion, must be perceived, not just unconsciously sensed, in order to be "authentic."

Whitehouse calls this perceptive awareness of one's own body movement, "kinesthesia," identifying it as a genuine sixth sense, and asks the question, "Could it be that the body is the unconscious, and that in repressing and, more important disregarding the spontaneous life of the sympathetic [and parasympathetic] nervous system, we are enthroning the rational, the orderly, the manageable, and cutting ourselves off from all experience of the [real] unconscious…which then take their revenge in the form of an exaggerated, compulsive fascination?"

Through Authentic Movement, the kinesthetic sense is first reawakened and then the body and the mind healed and developed. Said another way, through Authentic Movement, people can rediscover the parts of their bodies that are not felt, do not move and are not readily mentally available and in doing so, recover parts of their unconscious and conscious that have become inaccessible or dysfunctional. This implies that "something more" is involved in Authentic Movement than just body movement, active or passive. That "something more" is the *awareness* of the felt sense of the various body movements, which may, according to Reich, resultantly become "frozen."

Whitehouse's Authentic Movement involves relearning to move, connecting movements with the felt or kinesthetic sense of movement, the point being to heal the body to heal the mind.

Marian Chace pioneered the use of dance as a form of psychotherapy. Sharon Chaiklin and Claire Schmais, in "The Chace Approach to Dance Therapy" in the 1993 classic, *Foundations of Dance/Movement Therapy: The Life and Work of Marian Chace*, edited by Susan L. Sandel, Sharon Chaiklin and Ann Lohn, informed on page 76 that Chace, unfortunately, "never presented her material in a systematized manner." According to Chaiklin and Schmais, Chace regarded dance as a form of communication that uses four actions: (1) prescripted body actions; (2) symbolic moments; (3) the classical therapeutic relationship; and (4) rhythmic group activity.

Chace is said to have believed that distortions in body shape and movement were "expressions of maladaptive responses to conflict and pain," and that dance prepared patients to express their emotions. Both of these beliefs are intrinsically Freudian rather than Reichean, that is, that the body reflects one's mental attitudes, rather than creates one's mental attitudes. As such, Chace's ideas weigh heavily on the side of traditional psychotherapy, where dance, art, music, aroma, regression and talk therapies are primarily mental or "thought" (today, cognitive) therapies, their success being based on the direct expression of thoughts, assumed to be the necessary prelude to the resolution of physical signs and symptoms. Still, Chaiklin and Schmais, on page 78, state that Chace "made use of symbolic body action to communicate emotions and ideas that defy everyday use of language." Furthermore, "symbolism in dance therapy provides a medium by which a patient can recall, reenact and reexperience…the dance therapist utilizes this linkage by selecting appropriate dance images. For example, to help a patient who is holding back anger, the therapist may suggest the image of chopping down a tree."

Another fundamental difference between Whitehouse and Chace is that Chace would select and demonstrate movement responses designed to express to the client that "I know how you feel" or, more fundamentally, "I know what you're thinking." As she recreated the patient's behavior in her own body, she would sense what was "possible" and design further movements to help the client remember, reenact and reexperience.

Interestingly, Chace is said by Chaiklin and Schmais to recognize the importance of rhythm, music and song (but not necessarily costuming and visual representations) in a mostly eurythmic sense, primarily in a group context. In this sense, Chace's work mimicked classical "gestalt" psychology as developed in the 1940s and 50s by Fritz and Laura Perls. Again, however, the emphasis was on creating movements that would encourage clients to talk about their problems and through talking, resolve them—a distinctly Freudian rather than a Reichean approach.

According to Chaiklin and Schmais, Chace found that waltz music was one of the few kinds of music not disturbing to most clients; hence, waltzes were typically used to begin a group dance therapy session. Interestingly, ballroom dance, especially when danced socially with partners, has become a widely accepted part of the recreation programs of many mental hospitals. Ironically, Chaiklin and Schmais note that Chace is said to have held that modern jazz dance had "more value for mental patients than ballroom dance." This attitude proved formulative in the development of contemporary Dance Movement Therapy.

Chace's style of Dance Movement Therapy involves introducing body movements designed to help clients talk about their problems, the point being to heal the mind to heal the body.

American Dance Therapy followed and continues to follow Marian Chace's approach. That is, the emphasis is on the use of dance to support *psychologically-based* therapy (the emphasis is mine). Arguably the emphasis is likewise more Freudian, assuming that the body follows and reflects the mind. As an associate member of the American Dance Therapy Association (ADTA) since 2010 and an avid reader of the *American Journal of Dance Therapy*, I can say that American dance therapy generally reflects this thinking and has continued to develop primarily from the point-of-view of "modern dance" and gestalt therapy, the former rooted mainly in individual creative and expressive dance, and the latter rooted in the Perls' style of group action and "talk" therapy. One gets the sense that American Dance Movement Therapy is one of many developing forms of psychotherapy, dance being, like art in art therapy, a means to encourage talk (referred to in dance movement therapy as "communication"). One limitation of this is, of course, that most American Dance Movement Therapy is done in English, and as talking is a major part of Dance Movement Therapy, talking about psychological problems in English requires more than a basic knowledge of English. It requires quite a bit of skill to express nuances of thought and emotions. People for whom English is a second language or who speak little or no English, are significantly disadvantaged.

I've used English in addition to Japanese for over thirty years, at least half of my English use being American academic English in American colleges and universities. Talk therapy, as developed by mainstream psychologists, is highly dependent on not just a basic understanding and use of English, but often on particularly fine nuances. Consider the emphasis often placed on the Freudian slip, for example.

Furthermore, I studied dance beginning with partnered social dance, proceeding to keen partner amateur dance, to competitive and performance partner dance, rather than individual modern dance. One observation I've made in investigating and learning about Dance Movement Therapy is that even though the emphasis is on group dance, it emphasizes the individual dance rather than dance partnerships.

My background in therapy comes from massage therapy, a CAM therapy rather than psychology *per se*. Hence, I tend to look at Dance Movement Therapy more in terms of Whitehouse's approach. That is, the emphasis is on the use of dance to *support the body which in turn supports the mind* (the emphasis is mine). Arguably the emphasis is likewise more Reichean, assuming that the mind follows and reflects the body. Additionally, while contemporary American Dance Movement Therapy generally takes the point-of-view of "modern dance" and gestalt therapy, I believe there may be an alternative root embedded mainly in partnership and social dance, resulting in distinctive bodily and thereby mental benefits of this form of dance. Dance Movement Therapy, in this alternative sense, would be primarily directed at *actual body movements of dance partners* (the emphasis again is mine). One limitation of this is, of course, that such a Dance Movement Therapy approach, while freer of language constraints, would likely involve more touch, an issue over which American psychologists, educators and the public in general continue to express concern.

As a fellow of the American Association of Integrative Medicine (AAIM) in massage and somatic therapy, I began exploring the CAM therapies in more detail, searching for an approach to Dance Movement Therapy that better fit my interests and inclinations. In the process, I wondered if either European or Japanese Dance Movement Therapy organizations might be a better venue for me if either proved to be more heavily rooted in natural body movement than cognitive psychology. A cursory investigation of European and Japanese Dance Movement Therapy organizations looked promising; Japanese being my native language and my body of work drawing heavily from Eastern medicine and practices, I decided to join the Japan Dance Therapy Association (JADTA).

Setsuko Tsuchiya

Chapter 8
Japan and Dance Movement Therapy

Being from Japan, I feel a desire to see Japanese people benefit from Dance Movement Therapy. In fact, many Japanese are unaware of Dance Movement Therapy as a way to help resolve or, more importantly, prevent mental health problems. Part of the reason is that the basic concepts of mental illness, psychological counseling and dance as a mental health "treatment" are mainly Western. Furthermore, the dance movements in Dance Movement Therapy are often modeled on individual Western interpretive-style jazz and contemporary dance. My goal of language-free somatic therapy begged for a more social group form of dance more like social ballroom dancing in the US and festival-related bon dancing in Japan. Finally, Western Dance Movement Therapy often regards movement as an important prelude to talk therapy, where it is frequently assumed that the "real" therapy actually occurs.

For example, according to Chaiklin and Schmais, in their

article entitled "The Chace Approach to Dance Therapy" in San-del, Chaiklin and Lohn's book, *Foundations of Dance/Movement Therapy: The Life and Work of Marian Chace*, Chace recognized rhythm as important in organizing individual behavior and creating heightened feelings of strength and security, as well as develop solidarity between therapist and clients. In Chaiklin and Schmais' article, "The Chace Approach to Dance Therapy" in *Foundations of Dance/Movement Therapy*, the authors state on page 89, "the [dance] therapist elaborates...on a patient's symbolic movement expressions." In the same book on page 203 in "Opening Doors Through Dance" the important question, "Is the dancing curative?" is most succinctly answered: "This is not the function of dance therapy." The centrality of dance movement within traditional Western psychotherapy continues to be actively explored and argued within both the American and Japan Dance Therapy Associations.

Also, it is not entirely true that Dance Movement Therapy is based exclusively on individual, interpretive-style jazz and contemporary dance. For example, when describing the application of Dance Movement Therapy at St. Elizabeth's Hospital, Chace is said to have employed waltz, danced individually or as couples, eventually creating a "circle [group] dance" in which the tempo was slowly increased until the dance became more like a polka. Still, in "Techniques for the Use of Dance as a Group Therapy" on pages 205-206 of *Foundations of Dance/Movement Therapy*, it is stated that modern (by implication, individual, interpretive jazz/contemporary) dance sessions "have more value" in that they: (1) encourage the use of the entire body, rather than the feet alone, and (2) evoke more basic emotions. On the other hand, as a performance and competitive couples dancer, neither of these seem to me to be exclusive to modern individual, interpretive jazz and contemporary dance.

I can imagine a new style of Dance Movement Therapy (DMT), couples' DMT, which relies more on the experience of couples dancing together than the interpretations of a leader or dance therapist; that is to say, more *somatic* therapy than somatic *therapy*. Furthermore, in my opinion, couples' DMT holds great promise as not only a therapeutic approach, but also as an excellent preventive approach to mental health for Americans and Japanese alike. This is more in line with Reichean thinking.

In 1995, I read in a Japanese dance magazine called *Dance View* about a fledgling DMT effort in Japan. I was excited to read that a Japanese Dance Movement Therapist noticed that dance therapy, which was at the time just beginning to become popular in the US, had reached Japan.

According to the American Dance Therapy Association (ADTA), The National Board of Certified Counselors (NBCC) in the US began recognizing DMT as a mental health counseling specialty from 1998 to 2009, prompting the ADTA to adopt formal Dance/Movement Therapy training for certification. The Academy of Dance Therapists Registered (ADTR) certification currently offered by ADTA is now recognized by the Dance/Movement Therapy Certification Board (DMTCB) as the appropriate counseling specialty credential in DMT and is accepted by many states in the US as the key requirement for licensure. The important thing to note here is that DMT is herein recognized as a *counseling* therapy.

DMT quickly gained recognition in America. According to altMD online, "There are [already] over 1,200 certified Dance Therapy specialists in the US." This leads one to wonder why dance therapy wasn't initially as popular in other nations, for example, in my native country of Japan.

At this time, it is not easy to get a dance therapy license. In the USA, one generally needs a master's degree specifically in DMT. I searched the ADTA website as well as other sites and I found fewer than ten schools in the USA offering this specific master's degree. Of these, all emphasized the psychological over the somatic therapy.

The Japan Dance Therapy Association (JADTA), as well as other DMT associations throughout the world, appear to be watching and following the USA to see how the profession develops. At this time, JADTA doesn't require a license or master's degree. On the other hand, many outspoken Japanese Dance Movement Therapists turn out to have been trained in the USA, so it is likely that JADTA will continue to follow ADTA and eventually establish one or more schools of Dance Movement Therapy. Dance therapy is still largely new to Japan. What special value, if any, would DMT have for Japan, I wondered?

Japanese culture and society are, after all, quite different from American culture and society. There are five reasons why I think dance therapy isn't yet widely accepted and may never be widely accepted in Japan: (1) Japanese culture is a collective rather than an individual-based culture; (2) Families that have mental problems tend to hide them; (3) Japanese people generally don't seek a Western-style mental health counselor for their mental problems; (4) Western-style dance is still new to Japan; (5) Japanese people generally focus on sustaining longer, healthy lives rather than preventing or fixing mental health problems. Each of these differences, however, are also reasons why DMT, organized and presented differently, could become more widely accepted.

Japanese culture is a collective culture; almost everything is homogenous. Erica Rosen, a student at Washington University in St. Louis taking a course entitled Japanese Civilization, pointed out in her research paper, "The Influence of Culture on Mental Health and Psychopathology in Japan," published online in the 2001 edition of *Student Papers*, that if someone in Japan is in any way different or unusual, Japanese become uncomfortable. Dr. Yuko Kawanishi PhD, a sociologist specializing in social psychology and mental health at Tokyo Gakugei University and the author of *Families coping with mental illness: Stories from the US and Japan*, relates this in a more practical way on page 146 of her book: "Miyoko Tajima…heard someone talking behind her back, saying that because her son was (mentally) ill, she, the mother, must have some problems, too."

If someone has a mental problem in a Japanese family, the family often hides or covers the problem and pretends nothing has happened. Kawanishi points out that Japanese families prefer to use the term *shinkei suijaku,* which, loosely translated, means a "nervous breakdown," a vague phrase that implies a stress-related problem rather than a physical, mental or psychological problem. Specific terms for mental illness are, in fact, shunned in Japan. *Taijin-kyofu-sho,* or TKS, is another vague, general term unique to Japan that again indirectly implies stress-related illness, resulting in individual and family social withdrawal and public avoidance. These "diagnoses" and responses fit Japanese culture.

The Japanese have especially strong prejudices regarding mental illness diagnoses and therapies geared toward the elderly; it is important to remember that the Japanese, in general, respect, and in many instances, still venerate their elders. This is, therefore, a particularly important group in terms of needing a socially acceptable solution to mental health problems. It would be difficult to change the way the Japanese think about mental illness and therapy without appealing to the older generation first.

In America, people are more direct. They are more comfortable with accepting mental illness labels and usually seek specialized help for specific mental problems. Most American clients go to a therapist or counselor expecting to resolve their mental health problems. In Japan, if someone has such a problem, they commonly hesitate before going to a counselor. They are more inclined to struggle alone with the mental problem. Only if they're unsuccessful in their struggles do they generally decide to go to a hospital, and then, typically under a label or diagnosis that is not mental. Kawanishi says on page 148 that, "any illness related to the brain is regarded as 'insanity' in Japanese society. It is seen as the lowest kind of disease…Japanese family members are torn between their new and accurate understanding of the mental illness, love for the patient, and conventional social mores."

For the reasons above, I think Western-style DMT will be a challenge to establish in Japan. Getting therapy or having a counselor, even a "Dance Movement Therapist" is unusual and would likely be stigmatized. If someone mentions that he or she is seeing a "Dance Movement Therapist" or counselor, people won't want to be around the client and the counseling or therapy will have to be kept a dark secret.

On the other hand, Rosen states on page 7 of her paper that "while mental illness is seen as a stigma in Japan, physical illness is quite acceptable." This means that DMT, if publicized and viewed as health exercise, more physical than mental, should be more acceptable than mental health therapy or counseling.

DMT, on the other hand, based as it is on Western-style dance, would be relatively suspect to the Japanese. The Japanese are more used to Japanese-style dance and Eastern-style treatments like acupressure, acupuncture, Eastern-style massage or anma and Reiki treatment. These types of treatment help one not only recover, but, in the process, to feel more Japanese. Rosen comments that the goal of treating mental illnesses in Japan is to alleviate suffering by making the person more Japanese, and not necessarily by eliminating the underlying illness or disease, or learning to better understand one's self.

Furthermore, Japanese therapies are typically "quiet therapies," as they de-emphasize confrontation between therapist and patient like many Western mental health approaches. Instead, they typically encourage self-healing through meditation and self-reflection. Two examples of such quiet therapies are Naikan and Morita Therapy.

Naikan or Introspective Therapy, developed in Japan in the 1950s, is based upon Buddhist beliefs. Psychological problems are considered as manifestations of erroneous self-centeredness. The treatment is introspection for approximately one week in a medical hospital. A specialist, rather than a counselor, provides occasional guidance, if any at all, during this time.

In Morita Therapy, the patient spends one to two weeks in reflective and meditative isolation and is then gradually reintroduced to normal society. On page 13 of her paper, Rosen states that the goal of this type of therapy is to "make the patient yearn again for practical activity." Most Japanese people are coming to admit that Western medicine, in at least some areas, has progressed beyond Eastern medicine. However, if someone admits to a "psychological" problem, the Japanese still tend to view the person as morally or socially weak.

Finally, Japanese people today are living longer than any other race. In a 2009 article in *The Huffington Post* titled "Japan, San Marino Top Life Expectancy League," reporter Johanna Smith stated that according to the World Health Organization, the Japanese have the highest life expectancy in the world. The Japanese need a form of mental illness prevention and treatment that can benefit the growing elderly Japanese population and at the same time fit Japan's younger, emerging culture and society.

According to Nick Hurd, an American athletic trainer and writer interested in the health and aging of the baby boomer generation, bodies and minds weaken with age, but with specific exercises these processes can often be reversed. In an article entitled "What Exercises are Suitable for Elderly People...you Need to Know," on the online website Articlesbase, Hurd states the success of these specific exercises is limited by personal safety, and therefore, the exercises must be low impact and uncomplicated. In fact, aerobic capacity, muscle strength, balance, coordination, thinking and social skills are all part of, and enhanced by, dance. Certain forms of dancing, in particular social dance, incorporate low-impact movements that are appropriately strenuous, easier on joints, enhance balance and encourage coordination because one foot is always touching the floor. In such a case, there is maximal effect with less likelihood of injury. In addition, social dance is less complicated and strengthens individual thinking and social skills.

According to Clarke and Crisp, dance is among the most fundamental of human activities. There are many different types of dance, including religious, folk, ballet, tap, modern, country-western, jazz, ballroom, Latin and hip-hop to name just a few. When built on normal walking movements, dancing in any form is a fun and safe way to become and stay physically and mentally fit at any age. Latin dancing is particularly easy for both men and women to learn and is a great prelude to social ballroom dancing. Of all the different kinds of dancing, I believe that ballroom-style dancing is the most important to DMT because it also preserves and promotes healthy interpersonal couples' social interaction. Furthermore, ballroom-style dancing only requires proper shoes and a safe floor.

DMT seeks to help people express their feelings through body movement. For many Japanese, it is difficult to talk about feelings because people are not encouraged to show feelings like anger, sadness or fear. D. B. Givens, for example, in a 2009 on-line article, "Facial Expressions," posted on the Center for Non-verbal Studies website, cites Friesen, Morsbach and Ramsey as saying that while this situation makes it hard for Japanese people to talk about feelings or show affection through facial expressions such as smiles and laughter, they can and do dance to express their feelings. This is because expressing one's feelings through dance is not considered a sign of psychological or mental disease and therefore carries little, if any, social stigma. Furthermore, the Japanese have been taught that "natural" feelings, such as those expressed through dance, come from the heart and not the mind.

Japanese culture and society will become much more likely to accept Western-style DMT only if all of these ingrained cultural beliefs and behaviors change, something that would take years, if not decades or even centuries. This is especially so if DMT is considered a type of psychotherapy.

I can imagine the scope of DMT in the US eventually broadening to include couples social dance in addition to individual, interpretive jazz or contemporary dance movements. This is the key, I believe, to introducing DMT successfully to Japan in particular and the non-Western world at large. And I believe it to also be the key to understanding and applying *somatic* therapy internationally.

Setsuko Tsuchiya

Chapter 9
Should I Become an Albeit Unusual Dance Movement Therapist?

As I began investigating Dance Movement Therapy, I also began to rethink my life from four different perspectives: who I am; what life occupation I'm interested in; what my life goals are; and what additional education and training I would need to attain those goals.

Am I at heart, a Dance Movement Therapist? To find out more about who I am, I reexamined my life using a Jungian typology style test of common life values, Maslow's Hierarchy and Bloom's Taxonomy. Each helped me see myself in a slightly different way. When I examined the results of my life values inventory, I realized I am an independent thinker who's overly critical of myself. I never thought of myself as an independent thinker, but after moving to the USA and meeting my husband, I have had to become much more independent than when I lived in Japan with my family. I also found that since beginning my massage profession and college studies in the USA, I have become a more critical thinker in the American sense. I have always studied hard, but only recently have I become aware of all that critical thinking involves. In college, I wasn't ever sure if what I was learning about critical thinking was true—until now. I also think more about the value of my life these days.

When I first happened to read in *Dance View*, a Japanese dance magazine about Dance Movement Therapy, I imagined myself a Dance Movement Therapist. This idea intrigued me both as a competition dancer and a registered massage therapist, and these as it turned out, are both useful qualifications for becoming a Dance Movement Therapist in the USA or Japan.

At present in the USA, one generally also needs a master's degree in Dance Movement Therapy. However, when I further explored the ADTA website, I was disappointed to find that none of the fewer than ten schools in the USA offering this degree were located in Hawaii. More research revealed that no Hawaii colleges or universities were planning to offer this degree in the immediate future. That meant I would have to leave my family to pursue a master's degree in Dance Movement Therapy. In addition, existing programs generally stressed the psychological aspects of DMT rather than the somatic. These barriers, perhaps more than anything else, made me begin to challenge my ideas about myself and why I was pursuing DMT.

There were, I later discovered, two other possibilities: On the one hand, I could join the Japan Dance Therapy Association. With JADTA, I didn't need a master's degree in DMT because there was, as of yet, no prefecture or national license requirement. That isn't to say that Japanese Dance Movement Therapy hasn't progressed or isn't progressive. When JADTA began in 1999, there was only one level of therapist; since 2005, JADTA has introduced three: Dance Therapy Leader, Dance Therapist Associate and Dance Therapist. Actually, due to my competitive dance and massage therapist experience, I would be qualified to be a Dance Therapy Leader and since there is no license requirement, I could begin practicing in Japan immediately. If I registered as a JADTA Dance Therapy Leader and took some additional classes in Japan or the USA, I could likely qualify to be an ADTA-recognized Academy of Dance Therapists Registered (ADTR) Dance Movement Therapist in the USA through aggregate "grandmothering." There were, then, several pathways open to me.

My search to find out what life occupation I'm most interested in, however, ended up making me requestion my interest in Dance Movement Therapy, challenging me instead to widen my horizons.

DMT in the USA, as it presents itself, can be said to address the broader issues of somatic therapy about fifty percent of the time and psychological counseling the other fifty percent, and, while counseling in English might prove challenging but doable for a Japanese-born DMT for whom English is a second language, I suddenly wondered if I did become licensed in the USA exactly how effective I would really be at helping English-speaking Americans change their lives.

JADTA, as well as other DMT associations throughout the

world, appear to be following the USA and watching to see how the profession develops. While JADTA doesn't require a master's degree and a license isn't required in Japan, many outspoken Japanese Dance Movement Therapists turn out to have been trained in the USA, so it is likely that JADTA will continue to follow in ADTA's footsteps. Since dance therapy is still largely new to Japan and I am unsure what I could contribute to this profession in the USA, I decided to explore additional ways I might apply my own unique talents in this field. What specifically could I contribute then?

While my initial career goal was to be a professional Dance Movement Therapist in private practice in both the USA and Japan, what I came to realize is that I really wanted to develop a new style of DMT—couples DMT—with a much stronger emphasis on the somatic aspects. Given that this currently doesn't exist in the USA or Japan, I would have to establish it in both countries. In my opinion, such an approach holds great promise as an excellent physical and thereby mental health prevention and treatment modality for both Americans and Japanese, but especially for Japanese, as it would stress social-somatic issues rather than individual or group psychology.

According to ADTA, the National Board of Certified Counselors (NBCC) in the USA has recognized DMT as a mental health counseling specialty since 1998. In 2009, ADTA changed its name to the Academy of Dance Therapists (ADT). ADT now offers one level of certification: Dance Therapist Registered. When ADT became recognized by the newly formed Dance/

Movement Therapy Certification Board as the appropriate counseling specialty credential for Dance Movement Therapy, it rapidly became accepted by many states within the USA as the key requirement for licensing. Looking over ADT's training guidelines, I was again impressed with how much emphasis was being placed on psychological counseling *à la* Freud than somatic treatment *à la* Reich. In fact, looking over current and future training guidelines, it seemed to me as if somatic treatment was being valued more as a focus for generating counseling discussion, and if it continued to develop in the current manner would become even more so in the future.

Uncovering my own life goals and the education and training I would need to attain them were the greatest challenge. I knew that dance had to be a major element. However, there are many different types of dance. Add to these Dance Movement Therapy's regard of dance as a prelude to talk therapy and the position dance would play in my life became less, rather than more clear. It was then that I began to realize that any form of dancing built on normal walking movements is a fun and safe way to become and stay physically and mentally fit at any age. Dance Movement Therapy is currently based on individualized, interpretive jazz and contemporary dance movements, many of which are actually based on unnatural ballet-like movement like extreme high jumps (*batterie*), turns on the toes (*fouetté*), striking one body part with another (*frappé*), deep knee bends (*plié*), lifts (*relevé*) and splits. Of all the different kinds of dance, ballroom and Latin social partner dancing should be more appropriate because they are based on natural movements while at the same time preserving and promoting social interaction.

Furthermore, a couples social dance (CSD) model better fits the already existing United States' National Institutes of Health's CAM Body/Movement Medicine approach that requires specialized experience or certificate/diploma training rather than a psychology-related master's degree and license.

Of all forms of DMT, Japanese culture and society would be expected to accept DMT more easily if based on a modified CSD model. Once introduced to the USA and Japan, I would expect it to become a popular trend alongside the global excitement surrounding DanceSport and Olympic DanceSport, and eventually a cultural norm.

My occupational and life goals were clearly shifting from traditional Dance Movement Therapy as currently taught and practiced in the USA, to something broader and more fundamental with the emphasis on the body and partnership aspects.

Once my occupational and life goals became clear, so did my educational and training needs. To become a Dance Movement Therapist, using a CSD model, would require that I continue my social, performance and competitive dancing, delve deeper into the various CAM body therapies, and extract from it all a set of fundamental principles that when applied in any of these instances, would help resolve the problems of the body to help relieve the problems of the mind.

Initially, I hoped to simply expand the scope of DMT in the USA to include CSD based on natural movements in the CAM

Body/Movement sense, significantly changing its direction from that of primarily an individual or group modern dance-based prelude to psychological counseling. Furthermore, I thought to co-advance the idea and application of modified CSD to address prevention as well as therapy. This was the key, I believed, towards recreating, revitalizing, and reintroducing a more effective and appropriate DMT to Japan in particular, and in general to the USA and the world at large.

Setsuko Tsuchiya

Chapter 10
Another Look at Basic Natural Movement and Eurythmy

Almost everyone—from newborns to elderly—can move. In prehistoric times, people did so not only for utilitarian reasons, but also to communicate, play, exercise and tell stories. When human societies formed, people were said to have organized and developed these body movements into social dances for courtship, festivals and healing. Social dancing like this connects people with others and with nature. Some present-day churches even incorporate dance into religious prayer. In many cultures, dance is used to treat the sick.

Dance Movement Therapy, as one of the newer CAM therapies recognized by the United States' National Institutes of Health, uses body movements primarily taken from individual, interpretive jazz and contemporary dance, and applies them along with cognitive psychological therapy primarily to treat illnesses of the mind. It is important to distinguish right from the start between illnesses, which are *temporary conditions*, and diseases that have distinct causes or etiologies that if not treated medically or surgically, *would likely eventually lead to or directly result in death.*

The origins of Western dance go back to the ancient Greeks. Maurice Emmanuel, on page 9 of his classic 1914 book, *The Antique Greek Dance*, said, "the special qualities of Greek dance are a very keen sense of mimetic value, joined to perfect rhythm but somewhat lacking in precision." This is actually not a bad definition of modern dance. According to Emmanuel, sixth century B.C. Greeks danced their myths, history, sexual encounters, battles, even significant births and deaths at social events.

The Greeks used the word "eurythmy," a combination of the Greek words for *eu* or beauty and *rythmos* or rhythm, to identity the best and most appealing of rhythmic presentations that combined music, voice and dance; the term was used similarly by Greek and Roman architects to refer to perfect, harmonious visual proportions.

Eurythmy is rhythmically-integrated movement that brings together form, movement, words and music. Taken together, they are thought to reveal the essence of the world by creating a natural world language that allows for perfect expression. To the ancient Greeks, integrated rhythmic human movements and poetic-style music were particularly important.

In Rudolf Steiner's 1996 book, *A Lecture on Eurythmy*, eurythmy also embodied "visible" spoken words and letters to create a bridge between the living and their spiritual sources. For Dr. Margarete Kirchner-Bockholt, a Steiner-trained physician, in her 2007 book entitled *Foundations of Curative Eurythmy*, the essence of Steiner's visibly spoken words is the voluntary and involuntary movements involved in their production. When people move their bodies, including the muscles of their voice box or larynx rhythmically, mind and spirit are said to harmonize. The point here is that language or speech, whether social or talk therapy, is in essence another form of movement.

According to Emmanuel, the Greeks valued eurythmy more than anything else, even developing and applying philosophies in eurythmic terms. On page 35, he stated, "With the Greeks the dance was an art much more highly regarded than with us. The philosophers attributed to it a moral influence; they said that 'the dance is, of all musical arts, the one that most influences the soul'." On the same page Emmanuel also stated, "Plato said: 'It is the intermediary between the bodily rhythm and the soul, and it is the dance-gymnastic which teaches eurhythmy'."

During the Middle Ages, the Greek concept of eurythmia appears to have almost entirely disappeared from Western civilization, being broken by clerics and academicians into various components such as dance, music, fine arts, song, gymnastics, war, philosophy and religion. Gayle Kassing in his 2007 work, *History of Dance: An Interactive Arts Approach*, reports that each of these components was developed by church and secular "masters" into crafts, furthered by select heads of states, and performed for and taught to both the elite and the masses by professionals.

In 1919, Austrian-born artist, philosopher, scientist and educator Rudolf Steiner resurrected eurythmy as a path for personal and spiritual development as part of an overall effort he called "Anthroposophy." Through Anthroposophy, Steiner endeavored to reconnect these separate disciplines back to a holistic eurythmic from, in the process, developing one after another "natural," body-based eurythmic movement solutions for a wide variety of human problems. Steiner himself said in the C. Bamford translation of his 1994 book, *How To Know Higher Worlds - A Modern Path of Initiation*, that, in the process, he was attempting to reimbue the humanities with eurythmia. More important, according to an article posted on the Eurythmy Association of North America's organizational website, because eurythmy is based on rhythmic movements natural to human beings, everyone could participate and in theory at very least, join in this joyful form of fundamental human communication.

Eurythmy and eurythmics, however, were soon separated. Nowadays, eurythmics refers specifically to systems of learning and expression that employ body movement *à la* Steiner. One of the first modern eurythmic schools was created by Swiss music educator, Emile Jacques-Dalcroze, who in his 1920 work, *The Jaques-Dalcroze method of eurythmics*, described and incorporated both natural and unnatural (contrived, e.g. ballet) movements into his educational system.

It is important to distinguish between "natural" and "unnatural" movement, the latter in dance, reaching its zenith in French Ballet and more recently in the impressive and sometimes grotesque Canadian Cirque-du-Soleil-style of modern expressive dance. Emmanuel distinguishes this from "natural" modern dance, which on the other hand, is based on everyday walking, skipping, and running movements people use in normal life.

Hungarian dancer, choreographer and modern dance movement theoretician Rudolf Laban is generally recognized as the dominant pioneer in analyzing and recording natural (as well as unnatural) dance movements through his system of Labanotation according to Mary Clarke and Clement Crisp in their 1981 book, *The History of Dance*. However, while Laban is almost universally credited with being the originator, Clarke and Crisp also mentioned George Bickham, Jr., who, in a 1734 work entitled *An Easy Introduction to Dancing*, successfully employed simple figures, along with floor movement patterns and hand position diagrams to describe, convey, and archive normal dance movements. Since then, normal dance movements, including social ("partner") dance movements, have been further codified and refined by many, including Lillian Ray, Arthur Murray, Fred Astaire and the Imperial Society of Teachers of Dancing.

No work attempting to touch on "natural" dance would be complete without mentioning Isadora Duncan. Born in 1877, Duncan created and performed a primitive style of improvisational dance based on her recreations of what she thought to be ancient Greek dances. Duncan's aim, according to her 1927 autobiography, *My Life*, like that of Greek eurythmia, was to communicate universally through dance. She was known, for example, for appearing on stage barefoot, wearing a minimalist, diaphanous, Greek *peplos*, a one-piece wrap-around drawn at the middle. From these performances, a new type of "natural" or "natural improvisational" modern dance was born.

Duncan's contemporary, Ruth Dennis, according to Dr. Lynner Conner, Susan Gillis and Patrick S. Tse in their CD entitled *The Early Moderns*, was a modern dancer trained in ballet by Italian ballerina Maria Bonfante. Dennis added social dance forms and movements to Duncan's approach, making natural modern dance into something non-ballet trained singles or couples could do. Dennis performed as a skirt-dancer in a dime museum and later in vaudeville (Emmanuel explains that skirt-dancing is dance patterned after Ancient Greek dance that shows off the dancer's body movements through the manipulation of the skirt fabric). David Belasco, a famous Broadway producer and director, hired Dennis to perform her natural-body-movement skirt-dances with his company as a featured dancer, changing her name to Ruth St. Denis. St. Denis toured with Belasco's off-Broadway traveling production of "Zaza." Traveling to Europe exposed her to the work of several important European modern dancers and artists, including Japanese dancer Sado Yacco and the great English performer, Sarah Bernhardt.

St. Denis' artistic imagination was fired by Bernhardt's dramatic acting and Yacco's Eastern dance forms. Conner, Gillis and Tse point out that her personal goal changed to that of expressing emotion, especially that surrounding tragedy, in her dancing. By 1900, she was formulating her own theory of dance-drama which injected eurythmia solidly back into modern dance philosophy.

In 1914, St. Denis hired modern stage dancer Ted Shawn

and his partner, Hilda Beyer, to perform natural body movement communicative "ballroom dance" numbers. St. Denis watched, then performed "translations" of the dances. Shawn's popular, natural, movement-based couples dance rhythms included Ragtime and tango. Soon, St. Denis and Shawn became professional performance dance partners and initiated an era of natural movement-based popular ballroom and Latin couple dancing.

A third giant of contemporary eurythmic natural dance was Twyla Tharp. Born on July 1, 1941, Tharp is an Emmy and Tony award-winning American dancer and choreographer currently living in New York City. Tharp studied the natural partner dances of Ruth St. Denis and Ted Shawn, as well as those of Irene and Vernon Castle. Irene and Vernon Castle's natural couple dance approach to modern dance was used by Tharp to choreograph the popular Broadway play and later movie, *Ragtime*. Tharp later worked with famed modern dancer Mikhail Baryshnikov to incorporate pop music and natural contemporary dance forms into Broadway productions and movies. Oddly, as the online Academy of Achievement's "Twyla Tharp Biography" states, Twyla Tharp's most important contribution to Dance Movement Therapy, that of introducing natural couples dance music and movements as a form of somatic communication, is largely unacknowledged.

PREVENTION AND THERAPY

According to the 2007 *Dortland's Medical Dictionary for*

Healthcare Consumers, therapy is the attempted remediation of a health problem, illness or disease, and can be definitive, supportive or preventive.

In a 4 August 2010 personal communication, Dr. Daniel S. Janik, MD, a Fellow of the American College of Preventive Medicine and American Association of Integrative Medicine, related that definitive therapy for *disease* was for centuries, the sole province of physicians, while supportive therapy fell in the realm of health-related care and was the province of nurses, midwives and medical assistants. On the other hand, preventive therapy for diseases as well as definitive, supportive and preventive therapy for illnesses and common health problems typically remained in the hands of the common folk.

According to a 2006 article entitled, "Mental Health and the Legacy of Sigmund Freud," by Dr. Allan Schwartz, PhD, posted online on MentalHealth.net, and an online article by Dr. Leon Hoffman, MD, entitled, "The Interpretation of Dreams," posted on the American Psychoanalytic Association's online webpage and organizational postings on Child and Adult [Psychoanalytic] Training Programs, this situation changed in the mid to late 1800s with the development of psychoanalysis by Dr. Sigmund Freud. Freud, a medical physician, specialized in psychosomatic illness (neuroses) and mental diseases (psychoses). Freud, along with his associates and students, implemented psychoanalytic institutes throughout the world where non-physicians—called psychoanalysts—could learn the therapeutic principles of psychoanalysis and apply them to both illnesses and diseases. Most of the mental conditions they worked with were named by their physical attributes like hysteria and depression. Freud used the resolution of these psychosomatic attributes to measure the success of his new forms of therapy, including free-association, "talk therapy" and the interpretation of dreams.

Dr. Wilhelm Reich, a student and later colleague of Freud, argued that unreleased psychosexual energy, which he called "orgone" energy, produced physical blockages within muscles and organs that caused mental problems. According to Michel Cattier, in his 1971 book, *The Life & Work of Wilhelm Reich* and Janine Chasseguet-Smirgel and Bela Grunberger's 1986 work, *Freud or Reich? Psychoanalysis and Illusion* translated by Claire Pajaczkowska, Reich held that the physical act of sexual orgasm alone was an effective way to break through these blockages. Reich modified Freud's "talk therapy" to include touching patients to help increase their awareness of this tension and areas of blockages. In other words, he was redefining "talk" to include somatic communication. He began to ask patients to undress, initially partially, later sometimes entirely, before using talk, touch and/or controlled breathing to relieve these blockages. In fact, Reich closely observed his clients' natural body movements and reactions as a form of direct somatic communication in the process formulating natural physical interventions.

Reich's pioneering work using natural physical interventions that encouraged natural expression and thereby, a new kind of communication emanating directly from the body, set the stage for the development of the current wide range of body-based therapies collectively called by the United States' Institutes of Health, complimentary and alternative medical (CAM) therapies.

DANCE MOVEMENT THERAPY REDEFINED

While Wilhelm Reich's work was opening up new areas of body-based therapies like touch therapy, massage therapy and Rolfing, another of Freud's colleagues, Carl Jung, was developing a therapeutic technique he called "active imagination" to give his patients a better means of expressing subconscious thoughts through natural body movement. Joan Chodorow, editor of the 1997 book, *Jung on Imagination*, an edited collection of Jung's works, said in her introduction, "All the creative art psychotherapies (art, dance, music, drama, poetry), as well as Sandplay, can trace their roots to Jung's early contribution." Jung used dance with patients both as a means of personal expression and to "dance out their dreams."

After several years of Jungian analysis, professional dancer and psychologist Mary Stark Whitehouse blended active imagination with individual modern dance movements, which together she called Movement-In-Depth. Whitehouse saw deep psychological meaning in both natural and unnatural physical movements, a concept central to what she later called Authentic Movement. In my opinion, Authentic Movement has since remelded with individual modern improvisational dance, resulting in a number of popular Tai Chi-like forms that allow groups of participants to express and share individual feelings and emotions together in the tradition of Jung and Greek eurythmia.

It was the "first generation" of modern dancers, reported Dr. Robyn Flaum Cruz, PhD, ADTR, in her 18 October 2008 article entitled, "Perspectives on the Profession of Dance/Movement Therapy: Past, Present, and Future" in Wings of Support on The Bright Side website, who collectively pioneered Dance Movement Therapy. There was a strong desire by these early modern dancers to create a "feeling of community" and, through physical stimulation using dance movements, to encourage individuals to orally communicate thoughts, feelings, emotion. These first generation modern dancers, such as Isadora Duncan, Ruth St. Denis, Ted Shawn and Mary Wigman were followed by a second generation of modern dancers, including Martha Graham and Hanya Holm. All strongly believed that rhythmic movement allowed dancers to tap into and thereby better express deep, often unconscious emotions. This, coupled with an emerging appreciation of the therapeutic power of expressing emotion together with the modern development of body-based counseling psychology, led to the birth of DMT.

While all of this is undoubtedly true, I think that dance therapy was already being practiced when people first began freely using natural body movements for relaxation, enjoyment, health and healing, and later as an adjunct in the treatment of illness. Dance movement therapy was probably used to treat illnesses and diseases hundreds of years earlier, but these pioneers of modern dance were the first to define specific physical movements and mechanisms in which eurythmia was identified as important to communication and physical healing. Others soon began experimenting with using dance in body-based counseling psychology.

Sharon Chaiklin of the American Dance Therapy Association (ADTA) in an undated article entitled "Marian Chace: Dancer & Pioneer Dance Therapist" posted on the ADTA website, wrote that third generation modern dancer Maria Chace formally established Dance Movement Therapy as a distinct counseling therapeutic specialty. Chace was a visual artist who, after injuring her back, found it difficult to continue to practice the fine arts. Her attending physician suggested dance classes, a performing art, as a healing adjunct to medical therapy. As she healed, she changed her entire artistic focus to dance, eventually studying modern dance and choreography from Ruth St. Denis, Ted Shawn and other modern performance dancers working at the Denishawn School of Dance in New York City. Further influenced by the works of Carl Jung and Mary Whitehouse, Chace learned and developed her own philosophy of movement which she called Dance Movement Therapy.

Modern DMT incorporates elements of both eurythmia and humanistic counseling therapy. Dance, the most fundamental of the performing arts, is assumed to allow one to discover unconscious thoughts, feelings and emotions within him or herself using natural body movements, and to consciously reexperience them in the process through observation and reflection. When coupled with any of a variety of forms of "talk therapy," it came to be regarded as a powerful form of fundamental communication, and an especially effective medium for therapy. According to the National Coalition of Creative Arts Therapy Associations (NCCATA), "Membership/Working Groups" section, paragraph one, at NCCATA.org, DMT, a member organization of creative art therapists, is defined as "the psychotherapeutic use of movement as a process that furthers the emotional, cognitive social and physical integration of the individual."

Chaiklin in her previously cited article, "Marian Chace: Dancer & Pioneer Dance Therapist" relates that at the core of Chace's two-to-three-hour-long DMT sessions was circle dance. Chace treated patients, including combat veterans wounded in World War II, by assembling them in a circle and encouraging them to copy natural dance movements which she chose to help clients safely externalize their inner thoughts and feelings. She especially sought to foster individual awareness of any meanings that popped up during the copying of the rhythmic, heavily symbolic bodily expressions.

Maria Chace, Mary Whitehouse and later Trudi Schoop used modern dance movements to help groups of hospitalized patients recover from a variety of ailments more fully. In doing so, they created what many recognize as contemporary Dance Movement Therapy.

Dance Movement Therapy (DMT) in Europe

Venessa van Rensburg in a 2003 online article entitled "History of Modern Dance" posted on the South African National Society of Dance Teachers website, reported that throughout 1915, Ruth St. Denis performed with the USA-based Denishawn Dance Troop with her dance partner and later spouse, Ted Shawn, throughout Europe. Mary Wigman, a German modern dancer, found Ruth St. Denis' African and Oriental-style of modern dance inspirational. Wigman quickly developed a repertoire of solo, couple and group works incorporating the slower, longer rhythms of St. Denis' Eastern-influenced dance. Together with German modern dancers Rudolf Laban, Kurt Jooss and Herald Kreutzberg, Wigman spread pre-DMT modern dance throughout Europe. Unfortunately, this promising but fledgling movement came to an abrupt end when the National Socialist German Workers' Party seized power.

Mary Wigman, later in association with Francois Delsarte, Emile Jaques-Dalcroze and Rudolf Laban, founded the European school of modern dance, creating theories of body movement and expression as well as methods of instruction that eventually led to the development of modern European expressionist dance. Their theories and techniques quickly spread far beyond Europe to influence yet another generation of modern dance teachers and performers interested in DMT, and in the process, carried these theories and methods along with DMT to Russia, the United States, Canada, the United Kingdom, Australia, New Zealand and Japan. DMT today continues to spread throughout the world alongside modern dance, resulting in the establishment of national organizations of dance movement therapists, most reflecting the principles of ADTA and more or less incorporating eurythmia.

Dance Therapy Movement (DMT) in Japan

According to Mieko Fuji's 1998 book, *Mieko Fuji's Dance Therapy: Flexible Body and Refreshed Mind*, Fuji understudied Baku Ishii and Takaya Eguchi, both pioneers of modern dance in Japan. She also studied eurythmia under Sousaku Kobayashi, the first eurythmics teacher in Japan. In 1947, she opened the Fuji Fumiko Dancing Institute, taught modern dance and later, DMT.

The Reestablishment of Eurythmia through DMT

Several American journals of DMT currently exist, including the *American Journal of Dance Therapy*; *The Arts in Psychotherapy*; *Body, Movement & Dance in Psychotherapy*; *Journal of Physical Education, Recreation, & Dance*; *Moving On*; *Energy & Character* and *USA Body Psychotherapy Journal*, all investigating and directly or indirectly espousing the value of eurythmia through DMT.

Dr. Robert Sylwester at the 5 November 2007 meeting of the Neurobiological Learning Society in Honolulu, Hawaii, said that what distinguishes humans most is the extent to which we move. Sylwester related that humans move through the use of both body and language. Perhaps this is the essence of eurythmia and the very heart of eurythmic therapies.

The ancient Greeks held that eurythmy was perfect rhythmic

body movement to song and music. Nowadays, we hold eurythmia to also be a powerful way of expressing feelings. Even so, our understanding of eurythmia and eurythmic therapies, like Dance Movement Therapy, is still in infancy.

In short, DMT is affording the world a way to use eurythmia—natural rhythmic dance movement—to help people recover from as well as prevent illnesses and diseases, and in the process, rediscover a new, yet very old perspective: that of our spiritual meaning and place within the universe. After all, movement is a part of the very core of being human. Young or old, people enjoy moving their body. As a competitive performance dancer interested in Dance Movement Therapy, I like to believe that dance is life and life is dance, and that eurythmia once fully rediscovered, understood and correctly reapplied, will bring DMT back into holistic balance.

Chapter 11
The Basic Somatic Elements of Dance and Massage

Dance Movement Therapy is defined by the American Dance Therapy Association (ADTA) as the "psychotherapeutic use of movement to promote emotional, cognitive, physical, and social integration of individuals."

Furthermore, "Body movement as the core component of dance simultaneously provides the means of assessment and the mode of intervention for dance/movement therapy." Dance Movement Therapy, also called dance/movement therapy, is classified by the United States Federal Civil Service as a "creative art therapy" that includes art, dance, music and psychodrama.

Not everyone, however, would agree that dance/movement therapy is a creative art therapy. Interestingly, Naropa University and the International Somatic Movement Education and Therapy Association (ISMETA) consider dance/movement therapy a form of *somatic* therapy, and the United States' National Institutes of Health (NIH) National Center for Complementary and Alternative Medicine (NCCAM) on their website lists dance/movement therapy not under either Mind-Body Medicine or Manipulative and Body-Based Practices, but under Other Movement Therapies.

According to NIH NCCAM, movement therapies include a "broad range of Eastern and Western movement-based approaches used to promote physical, mental, emotional, and spiritual well-being." Examples include Structural Integration (Rolfing), a body-based practice that uses deep tissue fascial manipulation and movement education, and practices based on forms of energy and their internal movements (e.g. electromagnetic fields), putative energy (e.g. biofields) and energy fields (e.g. qi, ki, ch'i, orgone).

Somatic therapists, beginning with Wilhelm Reich, would also include DMT, massage therapy, Rolfing, acupressure, acupuncture and Reiki, all which have basic, fundamental tools, techniques, approaches and resources. The big question is exactly what they have in common that would further define somatic therapy *per se*. DMT can, for example, be considered one of the more recent offshoots of somatic therapy, featuring active dance movements as a specific form of energy movement. As such, all of the above as well as DMT, can be expected to have some basic, fundamental "movements" in common that are a part of somatic therapy's tools, techniques, approaches and resources that further uniquely define it.

Julie C. Van Camp, in her 2014 book entitled, *Philosophical Problems of Dance Criticism*, mentions that there are various definitions of a "dance movement" ranging from simple, rhythmic changes in posture and position to rhythmic patterns, to fundamental steps, to figures, to amalgamated figures and to routines as well. Dr. Daniel S. Janik, MD, PhD, a neurobiologist, in a 2015 personal communiqué, said to this list he would add kinesthetic feelings—the responses of smooth or "gut" muscles to physical stimuli or chemical emotions, as well as any resultant changes in body feelings over time.

So what are some basic DMT movements shared with somatic therapy? I recently emailed this question to the ADTA, which posted my question on their Research Forum on 9 November 2010 requesting an ADTA-registered or board-certified Dance Movement Therapist to respond. Unfortunately, no responses resulted. Internet searches for "basic movements" of "dance/movement therapy" did not yield any published, topically-relevant articles, even in the *American Journal of Dance Therapy* or *Body, Movement and Dance in Psychotherapy*, two major journals of DMT.

I also examined the Japan Dance Movement Therapy Association (JADTA) website and publication, *Japanese Journal of Dance Therapy*, and then proposed the same question I had asked the ADTA. This time, I received answers from a number of JADTA-certified dance/movement therapists, the gist of which is that there are no basic therapeutic DMT movements.

In general, DMT is about spontaneous client dance movements and mirrored therapist-selected dance movements. This means that any and all dance movements would be equally appropriate and by implication, of relatively equal therapeutic effectiveness. However, there are some dance movements, for example, ones that seem assaultive to the therapist or client, which could be said to definitely not be therapeutic. There is, then, the unstated implication that dance movements are more or less "situationally therapeutic," meaning some actually are more therapeutic than others, depending on the situation.

In a 1979 article by Sharon Chaiklin and Claire Schmais entitled "The Chace Approach to Dance Therapy" in *Foundations of Dance/Movement Therapy: The Life and Work of Marian Chace*, edited by Susan Sandel, Sharon Chaiklin and Ann Lohn, Chace is mentioned as having discussed particular movements used in group dance therapy by volunteer workers. These included basic walking steps and some figures from ballroom or social dancing. For example, some patients were "too sick" to participate in communal group sessions. Others proved unable to meet the demands of a changing group social situation. Still others experienced painful, difficult past experiences when assuming specific positions or executing specific movements. Shy patients especially found it difficult to tolerate a group ballroom dance class. On the other hand, severe, acute and chronic patients seemed to tolerate and respond to "modern" (free-style or spontaneous) dance or rhythmic movement group sessions. Furthermore, Chace and her students are reported to have used whole-body movements, rather than prechoreographed foot or arm movements or specific musical rhythms. Whole body movements were said to be of particular importance.

Another way to say this is that Chace didn't choreograph or record any specific movements, figures or routines. Her students, writing in Sandel, Chaiklin and Lohn's book, point out that Chace's collected papers also don't contain references or bibliographies. However, Chace refers to "basic dance" as the key to DMT "communication." She is also said to have referred to "basic dance" as having "basic principles." These include body action, symbolism, therapeutic movement relationship, and finally, rhythmic group activity.

As a part of body action, Chace was said to have analyzed "body distortions" associated with conflict and pain. She assumed that dance actions could help patients feel more relaxed and at the same time, stimulate them to express emotions. She is said to have strongly maintained that an important relationship existed between good posture and change in psychic attitude (which implies to me that certain basic postures are better than others). However, she also mentioned that in her practice, specific dance actions were determined mostly on a case-by-case basis.

Chace is further said to have purposefully used "symbolic body actions" to communicate emotions (actually, by strict definition, feelings) and ideas that defied verbal language. She is quoted as saying that "basic dance" is different from artificial and elaborate forms of dance used for entertainment rather than communication. She is also said to have said that dance actions associated with basic dance can "reproduce particular memories." Skipping and hopping, for instance, may induce specific memories from childhood. The implication here is that certain basic moments, often everyday movements or actions, can convey not only feelings or emotional content, but are linked to memories of past experiences and are therefore of particular importance.

Chace is also said to have discovered therapeutic movements that allowed her to relate visually and kinesthetically with her patients. Chaiklin says that Chace joined in her patient's behaviors, mimicking client movements, adding her own movement responses. This suggests to me that there are indeed specific, recognizable movements (Chace's "actions") that like specific verbal words, have specific somatic therapeutic meaning and value.

In their 1979 article, Chaiklin and Schmais mention that Chace is also said to have valued and used rhythm and rhythmic expression to communicate with and treat clients. Rhythm, to Chace, was "primitive" basic dance which included normal daily movements, actions and activities such as speaking, walking, working and playing to the rhythm of breathing or the pulse of the heart. In fact, Chace is said to have communicated that rhythmic expression is something reluctant patients can do with a particular sense of strength and security.

I believe that perceiving, copying or imitating breathing rhythms is probably one of the most basic "basic" movements or actions in both dance/movement therapy and by implication, somatic therapy. The sheer power of rhythmic breathing suggests it constitutes a basic somatic therapy movement.

Chace's four basic principles have been mentioned as principles of dance/movement therapy, and I believe, can be used to help further uncover and define additional basic dance and thereby, important somatic therapy movements.

According to Chaiklin and Schmais, Chace worked mostly with groups by mimicking patient movements and inviting patients to copy hers. But she also stated that she worked on occasion with individuals who needed more "direct contact." These clients were said to be too frightened, too demanding or too disruptive for the group. She described three kinds of such patients from a dance/movement therapy perspective: (1) manic, (2) depressed/psychotic and (3) schizophrenic. Each is described as having different characteristic movements and dance/movement therapy needs.

The manic patient is said to charge into space with exaggerated, quick movements that appear aggressive but are rarely directed toward another individual. Interestingly, she commented that they make exciting and stimulating dancers. While their natural movements are often strong and highly coordinated, they are interpreted as expressions of anger, destruction and despair.

Depressed/psychotic patients are said to be of two kinds: Depressed clients are sluggish, slow responding, indifferent to the environment, yet cognizant of his or her reactions. Psychotic patients are endlessly involved in unsatisfying activity.

Psychotic schizophrenics on the other hand, tend to withdraw from space and limit their movements to peripheral body parts like the head, feet or hands. In addition, the movements are just movements; that is, they are said to rarely communicate feeling or emotion. Leader and group expressions are largely ignored.

As Chace practiced her profession, she is said to have begun to notice that clients also had different short and long-range limitations and goals. She conceived these goals as addressing: (1) the therapeutic relationship, (2) individual body action limitations, (3) rhythmic group activity limitations and (4) key symbolic movements.

The Therapeutic Relationship

The long-term goal of the therapeutic relationship within DMT, according to Chaiklin and Schmais, is to reestablish client trust, independence and social awareness, while helping him or her come to accept social influences and ultimately, change.

Body Action Limitations

The long-term goal here is to help the client recreate a realistic self-body image, reactivate and integrate his or her various body parts, reconstruct a better postural gestalt, become more aware of inner sensations (feelings), mobilize energy, develop mastery and control of body movements and expand one's range of body expressions.

Rhythmic Group Activity Limitations

In this area of focus, the long-term goal is to help the client relearn how to project vitality, participate more meaningfully in shared experiences, channel energy within bounds, become aware of and responsive to others, to interact and bond with other people with disparate feelings and experiences and to develop an openness for new learning.

Symbolic Movements

The long term goal of Chace's final area of focus was to help the client integrate words, experiences and actions; externalize inner thoughts and feelings using the common, human, symbolic repertoire; recall the significant past; and resolve conflicts through insight and action.

In summary, Chaiklin and Schmais stated that Chace: (1) recognized the existence of "basic dance;" (2) understood that "dance actions" could help patients express blocked feelings and emotions; (3) held that a change in posture could cause a shift in psychic attitude; (4) recognized the singular importance of rhythmic breathing; (5) realized that some specific "dance actions," like chopping a tree, skipping or hopping, could lead some patients to suddenly recall incidents and events from their childhood; (6) identified that some "dance actions," like natural walking, included a powerful rhythmic component; and (7) said that sometimes rhythm could be shared even when clients were reluctant to imitate physical movements.

I conclude from all of this, that there are some movements of particular value to DMT and by implication, to somatic therapy, and that conversely, not all movements or rhythms are beneficial. I was sorry to learn that Maria Chace didn't explicitly identify, nor did her students or students' students recognize the existence of basic movements that are of special benefit.

Recalling the importance Maria Chace placed on posture and postural reintegration, I emailed Linda Webber at the Rolf Institute regarding the basic movements involved in therapeutic posturing (in dance, this would loosely mean "center" and/or "frame"). I thought that Rolfing, an NIH-recognized CAM therapy based on psychologist Dr. Ida Rolf's techniques of postural reintegration, might lend a clue as to some further basic movements. Mr. Robert McWilliams, Certified Advanced Rolfer, Rolf Movement Practitioner and Master of Fine Arts in Dance, emailed me back and said that Rolfers consider the following as "key" movements: (1) breathing, (2) standing erect and (3) walking in a balanced, coordinated fashion.

The basic movement therapies used on the Rolfing table varied depending on the client's abilities and how well their body adapted to Rolfing movement, but special emphasis was always placed on deep breathing through the shoulders, ribs, hips and legs. At the same time, key observational questions might be, for example, does the client fixate on inhalation or exhalation? Is there an underlying holding pattern to the client's "breathing?" What about breathing rhythm in stance and gait? Are they able to "drop down" (let go of individual movement idiosyncrasies) while on the Rolfing table? The idea of rhythm and pacing come up yet again if the client's situation involved trauma—unwanted life or for that matter, therapeutic interventions "too much, too fast, too soon." Rolfers, like DMT therapists, frequently attempt to identify, focus on, bring to consciousness and at times match a client's intrinsic breathing rhythm for a variety of reasons.

Regarding standing posture, typical observational questions include: How well can this person balance on their two feet? Does he or she demonstrate a strong enough base of support to allow a relaxed stance and/or gait? Is there spring and balanced ease in their step? How well can the client use his or her feet, legs and hips to funnel ground force upwards and distribute weight down and outwards?

Regarding gait, observational questions include: How free is the client, in general or in specific regions of the body, to fully flex and extend muscles, to reach into space, to oppose or yield to gravity? Does he or she act as if having no backbone, or does the client give an impression of three-dimensional spatial full-ness—a perceived sense of projected height, width and depth?

According to McWilliams, in Rolfing these observational questions illustrate the "primary elements" that a Rolfer will work with. It was interesting to me that there was overlap with DMT, Rolfing and massage therapy, and that all of these primary elements mentioned speak directly to the body rather than the mind.

Rolfing operates on the premise that someone who is more relaxed and secure physically will benefit psychologically and emotionally. Regarding past traumas, contemporary Rolfing training teaches Rolfers to also attend to the physiological signs of "trigger activation" in clients, and to respond appropriately on a *somatic* level (the emphasis is mine).

I think that much of the work Rolfers do stimulates or calms unwanted, conditioned, traumatic reflexes that have been acquired by the body. As a medical massage therapist and dancer, I can think of specific somatic triggers, for example, in the bottoms of the feet, or the lumbar triangle, either of which might interfere with normal leg movement. I don't know if that was exactly what Dr. Ida Rolf had in mind; however, I am impressed that Rolfers hold the primary elements of breathing, standing and walking in the same regard as Marian Chace apparently did.

Returning specifically to Japanese DMT, Mieko Fuji, in her 1998 book, *Mieko Fuji's Dance Therapy*, stated that movements that concentrate in the Tanden, Dantian, Dantien or Tant'ien chakra, (the Manipura or Navel chakra), are particularly important, as they involve meridian-based energy flow induced movements that can help a client move more easily and release any trauma-related tension from nerves, muscles and tendons. Hand movements, either active or passive, especially help reestablish deep breathing and allow ki, qi and chi energy to flow more freely. While this distinctly "Eastern" style of identifying and describing key basic movements may sound odd to Westerners, previously quoted Janine Chasseguet-Smirgel and Bela Grunberger in *Freud or Reich? Psychoanalysis and Illusion*, informed that Wilhelm Reich, the "father" of Western somatic therapy, spent much of his life researching energy in the form of "orgone" energy. He believed, however, that this energy was not necessarily confined to meridians or the body, but could be found everywhere, inside and outside of the body. If alive today, I think that Reich would say that if a person can free this energy, he or she would acquire a better balance in their movements and thereby thoughts. This is, I believe, what DMT is grappling with and trying to state: Manipulating the body allows release of tension or stress, and there are key manipulations, like effective breathing, some active, some passive, that underlie DMT and all somatic therapies as a whole.

In summary, my understanding of basic body movements for dance/movement therapy is that they are neither commonly acknowledged, recognized nor understood. While difficult to define, the basic dance movements involved directly or indirectly in deep breathing are clearly of particular importance. Next in importance are posture, walking, skipping, running and jumping in a kinesthetically communicative manner to an intrinsic rhythm, especially a socially-acceptable, mutually-shared rhythm. I also believe that through continued careful, gradually refined observation, a set of better-defined basic movements will emerge. One of my challenges in life will be to progress this further.

Setsuko Tsuchiya

Chapter 12
Progressive Muscle Relaxation

During massage and my investigations into body/movement therapy, one issue consistently came up: tight and sore muscles. Not necessarily pain in the strictest sense, but muscles that displayed less than full range of motion and often hurt when actively stretched or passively kneaded and stretched. Dr. Edmund Jacobson MD, in his book, *Progressive Relaxation*, refers to this as "muscle tension" when it occurs in persons who ordinarily would not necessarily be called "nervous." Some psychologists like Dr. Peter A. Levine PhD in his groundbreaking book *Waking the Tiger—Healing Trauma*, call it "frozen residue of energy" in the tradition of Dr. Wilhelm Reich.

This tension or energy is commonly thought to be relieved by rest; however, Jacobson and Levine both agree that rest actually does not release this kind of tension. Instead, the blocked energy and resulting muscle tension remain frozen in the body, causing psychic distress, expressed globally in terms of post-traumatic symptoms or post-traumatic stress disorder. In fact, this tension has been attributed as both muscle (somatic) and nerve (somatic and/or psychic) tension. In either case, the common de-nominator is muscle tension. Levine states on page 176 of his book, "Unfortunately, humans often do not completely discharge the vast energies mobilized to protect themselves [during a trau-matic event]. Thus…they…experience often terrifying and com-pulsive flashbacks."

Jacobson, on page 219 of *Progressive Relaxation*, explains it this way: Emotions involve hypothalamic and cortical centers but also peripheral localities, including all types of muscles. It seems most likely, according to present knowledge, that the subjective experience of emotion (that is, the perception of the whole body reaction to a change in circulating chemicals, commonly referred to as "hormones") is largely derived from muscular proprioceptive impulses (more specifically referred to as "feelings"). In essence, muscular elements (feelings) appear as a result of different emotions (circulating chemicals). Relaxation, therefore, would be the opposite state.

Furthermore, Jacobson continues, "Certain tests suggest that if the outward manifestations of emotion are suppressed or con-cealed by the individual, the affective phenomena [feelings] are all the more increased." In other words, "subjects report that the emotional experience diminishes, disappears or fails to appear," and by failing to appear, the result would be similar to Levine's "frozen residue of energy [unexpressed or unperceived feelings]." But, where in the body does this "residue" reside? Reichean psy-choanalysts Janine Chasseguet-Smirgel and Bela Grunberger clearly state on page 178 of their previously mentioned book, "emotions, affects and character defenses come to be inscribed in our bodies," adding, "people who practice massage, especially those with psychoanalytical training, would fully agree with this idea." But where specifically within the body do they reside?

Jacobson says that the emotional residue, as frozen energy or tension, resides within the body's neuromuscular system, including both striated ("voluntary" skeletal) and smooth ("involuntary" organ) muscle tissues. Releasing this muscular tension, which Jacobson calls "relaxation" (in the strictly muscular sense), is the goal. Levine at first seems to disagree, stating that relaxation "is not the answer" on page 29 of his book, but, I believe he is referring here to general relaxation or relaxation that results in the dropping of one's mental defenses and subsequently reliving the trauma. The goal of relaxation, then, is to relax specific tense muscle groups in small increments—just enough to release some of the frozen energy, but not enough to tip the individual into re-experiencing the original trauma, which, if allowed to occur, would simply compound the person's overall tension.

This residual energy will not simply dissipate or "go away" of its own accord. Rather Levine on page 20 states, it "forces the formation of a wide variety of symptoms." Jacobson implies this when he states that relaxation of one muscle group tends to affect a similar condition in other muscle groups. The goal, according to Jacobson, is neuromuscular reeducation—by releasing a tense muscle group in small increments, over and over, to create a new "felt sense" or "feeling" when the muscle group is subsequently contracted.

Both Jacobson and Levine agree that it is this felt sense which must be readjusted or reeducated. Felt sense can be distinguished from emotion (the presence of a circulating chemical in the blood that results in one or more feelings) and "feelings," which involve sensing and perceiving a muscle or muscle group's tension.

Felt sense has proven challenging to define in words. Levine quotes Eugene Gendlin from his 1981 book entitled, *Focusing*, as stating it "is not a mental experience but a physical one...a bodily awareness of a situation or person or event." I prefer the simpler definition of a feeling as conscious awareness of muscle *tension*, to distinguish it from a more general thought, perception or emotional state.

This distinction is important. For example, in traditional psychological therapy, suggestion, the placebo effect and cognitive realization through verbalization, called collectively "talk therapy," are considered to play a major role in resolving anxiety. In somatic therapy, talk therapy, as such, plays a minor role. In fact, Jacobson suggests that during muscular reeducation, no technical suggestions be given orally and to keep distracting verbal communication between therapist and client to an absolute minimum. Furthermore, before a period of therapeutic relaxation, it is recommended that the client "avoid discussion of any topic," focusing his or her attention on bodily sensations rather than thoughts. Given these observations, one can think of the felt sense (feelings) as internal body sensations, which are the fundamental concerns of contemporary somatic therapists. As such, posture, breathing, pain, temperature, swelling, tenseness, irritability, position and movement through space and time all become important issues for the somatic therapist. In addition, Jacobson and Levine both hint strongly that rhythmicity is also important.

In chapter five of his book, *Progressive Relaxation*, Jacobson states that the aim of therapy is to train the patient to treat him or herself in order to become free of the need for a therapist. The client is discouraged from learning and memorizing what muscles are responsible for various movements, but rather be acutely aware of their tenseness. Even so, Jacobson admits that developing a muscle-sense is not easy or always successful.

A particular advantage to progressive muscle relaxation is that clients can learn to progressively relax individual muscle groups while sitting, reading or even going about one's work. The effect of doing individual muscle group relaxation is that it has an overall calming effect on the rest of the body as well as the mind. This specifically fits Reich's concept of healing the body to heal the mind. On page 188 of *Progressive Relaxation*, Jacobson states, "with progressive muscular relaxation…[obtrusive] recollection, thought-processes and emotion gradually diminish." Furthermore, as emotions subside, the individual completely relaxes all striated muscles. When a client is completely relaxed in this manner, previously bothersome emotional states typically fail to exist. It is also important to note that throughout all this, suggestion plays a minor rather than a major role.

Jacobson wrote not only *Progressive Relaxation*, a book for professionals, but *You Must Relax*, a book for non-professionals.

In *You Must Relax*, Jacobson decries today's highly competitive society and the resulting individual's compulsive need to prove him or herself through excessive effort, citing muscular tenseness, for example, as a consequence of wives and husbands being increasingly unable to agree. In response, their children, both at home and school, acquire their own body tension through constant observation and elevated emotions. This, says Jacobson, is reflected in a sense of general fatigue and failure to sleep well, a condition not unlike that which psychologists call "depression." Headaches, especially in the back of the neck and shoulders, constipation typically accompanied by diarrhea, burning sensations in the upper abdominal area often reflecting the presence of stomach or duodenal erosions or ulcers, angina pectoris (chest pain from coronary insufficiency), asthma, joint pain from chronic osteoarthritis, dysmenorrhea (pain on menstruation), dyspareunia (pain or discomfort with sex), are all characterized by measurable neuromuscular tension, and are often said to be psychosomatic in origin. In addition, smoking can be considered a sign of unconscious or conscious suicidal intent, and use of alcohol considered a sign that the client is attempting to block unwanted or uncomfortable memories. Tranquilizer use can similarly be considered a sign that the client's physical and emotional defenses are no longer able to prevent him or her from reexperiencing the effects of chronic stress and/or past traumas. On page 10 of *You Must Relax*, Jacobson states there is consistent evidence that "the success of any form of present-day psychiatric treatment...can be measured by decline of tension states in the neuromusculature." Another way of saying this is that there is "no psychic occurrence in man which is non-somatic." That is, everything psychic has roots in the body.

Interestingly, Dr. Daniel S. Janik stated in a recent personal communiqué that in his experience, "depressed" clients are not really neurologically or muscularly "depressed." In fact, they are neuromuscularly hyperactive, in Jacobson's words, "spending too much energy" trying to suppress intrusive feelings, hence, the word "relaxation" is most properly used to mean discontinuance of all voluntary and most nonessential involuntary muscular contraction. One can say that making an effort to relax is in itself a failure to relax. One can also say that in conserving neuromuscular energy, one conserves not only bodily reserves, but also resulting mental reserves.

According to Jacobson in *You Must Relax*, traumatic events are commonly the basis of stress, both acute and chronic. Acute stress, the "fight or flight" reaction everyone experiences following a traumatic (i.e. unwanted) event or occurrence, is short-lived and protective. However, if the source of stress or stresses continues for more than a few minutes, acute stress turns into chronic stress, which may persist throughout one's life and be destructive to the body, and as such, the mind. I would point out here that "trauma" is being used in the strict sense of any unwanted event or occurrence.

Jacobson states on page 47 of *You Must Relax* that "scientific relaxation is not just lying down or sitting up in quiet manner with good intentions. It is as technical an undertaking as running a plane." Furthermore, as stated on page 49, "physical exercise has little relationship to technical relaxation." In essence, technical or "real" relaxation is the absence of striated or "voluntary" muscular activity. In fact, "it seems necessary to the patient to learn to recognize when and where he is tense during fears and to relax the localities involved [in order to resolve the fears]," Jacobson states on page 53.

It is then, not enough to just generally "relax." In fact, Jacobson's progressive muscle relaxation refers to relaxing specific muscles and muscle groups progressively. The first effort is therefore directed at identifying specific muscles and muscle groups that are tense. This is not so difficult for a massage therapist who can feel a client's muscles beneath his or her fingertips. It is commonly much more difficult for the client, however. For example, one may have tenseness in the muscles of speech, the muscles of eye movement or the forehead ["persistent frowning" or "age (worry) lines"]. On the other hand, it is equally important to identify those individual muscles associated with a client's felt sense of tenseness, especially those associated with fears or anxiety.

Jacobson relates the importance of not only the therapist, but also the client observing and identifying individual tense muscles, the ultimate goal of progressive muscle relaxation being for the client to no longer need the assistance of the therapist.

Of equal importance is the objective assessment of muscle relaxation. Jacobson reported using quantitative action potential recordings to do this. Most therapists, however, won't have a physiology research laboratory at his or her command. To measure success, Jacobson suggests that therapists use a combination of client and therapist observations regarding the slow but continual comparative change in specific muscle tension over time. Another useful but more qualitative test is quality of sleep. Jacobson claims this can be objectively assessed using tendon reflexes. For example, he relates that during "tense" sleep, a freely hanging leg kicks vigorously when the tendon below the kneecap is tapped with a reflex hammer. In deep, "relaxed" sleep, the kick is significantly less or absent altogether.

But relaxation in somatic therapy terms means more than a sense of relaxation. A pleasant vacation, for example, may not always prove relaxing. In fact, it is often the opposite. It is impossible to not be physically and mentally relaxed if all the voluntary striated muscular components are completely relaxed. That is, relaxation as defined here is a purely muscular phenomenon. Any felt sense of muscular relaxation or overall sense of body relaxation is the result of individual muscles being relaxed. Interestingly, Jacobson states that if one relaxes skeletal muscles (voluntary striated muscles over which one typically exercises control), corresponding internal smooth muscles like heart, airway and gastrointestinal muscles tend to likewise relax.

According to Jacobson, the "progressive" in progressive muscle relaxation involves three "aspects": (1) the client relaxing a muscle group, for instance, the muscles that bend the right hand, more and more over time; (2) as the client learns to relax the muscle group, he or she learns to discriminate the various individual muscles in the muscle group and becomes able to relax them individually, one at a time, even more over time; and (3) as the client learns to relax individual skeletal muscles, he or she begins relaxing corresponding smooth muscles, resulting in a felt sense of repose. This sense of repose results from release of the energy being used or blocked by the skeletal and smooth muscles. By this, I take it to mean that the body's resting energy is no longer as regionally intense due to blockages, but free to flow and be used throughout the body.

This brings us to the fundamental nuts and bolts of progressive muscle relaxation, that is, how exactly to do it. Jacobson relates in both *Progressive Relaxation* and *You Must Relax* that it is not really that difficult to learn to relax in the somatic sense. On page 164 of *You Must Relax*, he states: "To clarify this matter, stretch out your arm and lift a heavy weight with it. As your muscles contract, you find yourself exerting effort; you find that the lifting is difficult. But suppose that you do not bother to lift the weight, just letting your muscles relax. This is the negative of exertion, the negative of difficulty...many persons have acquired habits of exerting themselves in everything they do [including relaxing], so that they contract some muscles...even in trying to relax." Jacobson calls this "effort error," which he says must be eliminated in order to achieve "real" muscle relaxation. He also states that effort error is what distinguishes true muscular relaxation from exercise or "forced" relaxation.

To begin progressive muscle relaxation, Jacobson suggests a quiet room with a comfortable couch or bed, sufficiently wide for the arms to lie on either side without touching the body. The client lies prone, facing the ceiling. Jacobson suggests touching the fingers of one of the client's hands lightly with a wisp of cotton to help focus attention on the underlying area. Next, the client is instructed to let the hand and fingers become totally limp, then to tighten them slightly, and again let them become totally limp. In this way, the client begins to distinguish between effort error and total relaxation. Once a muscle tension baseline has been established, the client is instructed to tighten the muscle or muscle group ever so slightly, breathe deeply and then release both breath and the muscle or muscle group completely. It is important, Jacobson states, to distinguish between release and making an effort to relax the muscles. That is, "every effort to relax is [a] failure to relax," which emphasizes the importance of releasing all control and tension in the muscle or muscle group rather than "making the muscles relax." Jacobson recommends three such episodes during any hour of "practice," stating that the best results are obtained if the total period, whether led by the therapist or client, lasts about two hours. This represents the basic format for progressively relaxing all skeletal muscle groups and later all individual skeletal muscles. Jacobson specifically warns against the use of mental exercises, like mantras, stating on page 189 of *You Must Relax*, "At no time should you make an effort to stop thinking or to 'make your mind a blank'. Throughout your course, your sole purpose is to relax muscles progressively, letting other effects come as they may."

Beginning with muscle groups, he, for example, recommends helping the client recognize and relax the muscle groups in one area before moving on to another. A possible course would be to begin with one arm, followed by both, followed by the back and neck, followed by the legs, and finally chest and abdomen. Once this course is accomplished and the client can relax the major muscle groups him or herself, one can focus on relaxing "steady tensions" inherent, for example, in posture, breathing, eyes and eyelids, reading and conversing. The same basic format is used, directing effort at relaxing skeletal muscles and allowing the corresponding smooth muscles to relax. It is important, Jacobson relates, to also attend to "differential relaxation," that is, the ability to relax the muscles during exercise, including "dancing relaxation."

Jacobson's pioneering work in somatic therapy has recently been further augmented by Dr. Peter A. Levine's Somatic Experiencing® approach.

Chapter 13
Waking the Tiger—Healing Trauma

Dr. Peter A. Levine, in the acknowledgement section of his 1997 book entitled *Waking the Tiger - Healing Trauma*, states, "I am profoundly indebted to the legacy of Wilhelm Reich, whose monumental contribution to the understanding of energy was taught to me by Philip Curcurruto, a man of simple wisdom and compassionate heart."

Levine, on page 19 asserts, "It's all about energy." Not just Jacobson's muscle tension described above, but in the special sense of specific residual muscle tension after trauma. Traumatic symptoms, he states, "stem from the frozen residue of energy that has not been resolved and discharged; this residue remains trapped in the nervous system where it can wreak havoc on our bodies and spirits. The long-term, alarming, debilitating, and often bizarre symptoms of PTSD [Post Traumatic Stress Disorder] develop...in, through and out of the 'immobility' or 'freezing' state."

Levine discusses the example of a running impala about to be killed by a lioness. It is, he explains, the difference between the inner "racing" of the nervous system and the beast's sudden physical immobility that creates a "forceful [energy] turbulence." It is out of this tornado of energy that the symptoms of traumatic stress are said to emerge. In essence, energy flow is blocked. In order to resolve the symptoms of the traumatic event, the blocked energy must be remobilized. This blocked energy, when properly mobilized, can resolve physical symptoms and thereby mental duress. Levine, like Jacobson, says that relaxation (in the general sense), exercise, meditation and emotional catharsis (e.g. mentally reliving the traumatic event) are not sufficient to unblock the trapped energy. In fact, given the client's unconscious propensity to try to reenact various aspects of the trauma to bring it to consciousness, resulting traumatic repetitions can often result in retraumatization, compounding the original physical and mental signs and symptoms.

Levine's approach to unblocking this energy is a careful, gradual release called Somatic Experiencing®. It is important here to state that Levine's Somatic Experiencing® does not necessarily involve any mental or even, for example, shamanistic reexperiencing. It is primarily somatic.

On page 63 of *Waking the Tiger*, Levine gives an example in which a client repeatedly exposes his or her body to pulsing water. "Put your full awareness into the region of your body where the rhythmical stimulation is focused…pay attention to the sensation in each area, even if it feels blank, numb, or painful," Levine states. At the beginning of the healing process, Levine holds, one must *experience* as a prelude to perceiving and recognizing this kind of felt sense. According to Levine, the physical senses of sight, sound, smell, touch and taste represent an important portion of the felt sense, but it also includes related consciousness of the body's internal awareness, for example, body position, muscular tension and involuntary movements. It isn't important to interpret, analyze or explain what is happening, only to consciously experience the "felt sense," in an effort to reawaken it from its frozen state. Experiencing any one of these sensations as a felt sense is a beginning point.

As one progresses, felt sense extends to include subtlety, variety and rhythmicity. The felt sense can then be experienced not only as a static event, but within the broader context of the body's own intrinsic rhythmic/cyclic events. Becoming aware of biological rhythms opens the door to awareness of heartbeat, breathing and changing moment-to-moment hormonal cycles which in turn, unlock emotions. This process will happen if the client is willing to explore not only the sensations, but the resulting feelings, that is, the felt sense of muscles contracting, which accompany somatic experiencing. On page 83, Levine states, "you can't push the river. Becoming attuned to these rhythms and honoring them is part of this process."

According to Levine, in today's world most people lack the ability to stay present to the nuances of their external and accompanying internal "landscapes." But what is it exactly that such people are not "in tune" with? On page 111 of *Waking the Tiger*, he states, "The forces underlying the immobility response and the traumatic emotions of terror, rage, and helplessness are ultimately biological energies." "Renegotiating" traumatically learned events requires a step-wise approach in which the felt sense is used to gradually locate, contact and mobilize the trapped energy. For many victims, arousal (awareness of feelings and the emotions that underlie and accompany them) are initially inseparably linked to the immobility response—terror, horror, rage and helplessness. But the drive to resolve trauma can be as powerful and tenacious as trauma's symptoms.

Levine points out on page 176 that, "Unfortunately, humans often do not completely discharge the vast energies mobilized to protect themselves. Thus, when they enter the second phase, they are reviewing the event, but remain in a highly aroused state. This heightened energy level will not allow the 'playful' reviewing to occur. Instead, they may experience often terrifying and compulsive flashbacks." That is, without proper preparation and approach, one is subject to reliving the various parts of the initial event and being retraumatized.

To Levine, "renegotiation" and "transformation" of the trauma require specialized Somatic Experiencing®. This specialized form of somatic therapy is all about moving blocked energy in small increments until the client is able to reexperience the traumatic event without resulting energy reblockage. Most cognitive psychologists tend to focus more on the "talking therapy" portion, but, in the end, it is all about the client's own ability to ground and stay grounded without exerting special effort. That is, it is about free energy flow.

Levine's description of Somatic Experiencing® reminds me

how important grounding and the free flow of energy is to every-day life. Dance, for example, involves "springiness" which is in effect, the ability to rhythmically ground, "unground" and re-ground. In couples dance this is sometimes referred to as "smooth" or "gooey connection"—the flow of energy from one partner to the other and back. Such energetic freedom is immediately apparent after successful massage or progressive muscle relaxation. Empowerment, the final step in all forms of somatic therapy, is about the client being able to freely move energy for him or herself without a therapist or guide. If there is one particular difference between somatic *therapy* and *somatic* therapy it is the former's reliance on the formation and maintenance of a dependency relationship. With this comes issues of transference and counter-transference. The power of *somatic* therapy is that it speaks directly from body to body and doesn't depend on either talk or dependency. Clients are *from the first* directed to become independent of the therapist and in control of their own energy movement and, ultimately, recovery. One final comment before leaving Somatic Experiencing®: Transference and counter-transference, major issues which can result in further damage to clients, don't seem to be major issues in *somatic* therapy, unless of course, one takes it to a Reichean extreme with inappropriate sexual energy mobilization and release.

Setsuko Tsuchiya

Chapter 14
In Search of Somatic Therapy

Lucy...her right arm in a sling, overwhelmed and exhausted from being in acute pain...had re-injured an old rotator cuff tear in the right shoulder...in constant pain, [she] couldn't sleep, couldn't work, and needed some relief. The husband was a massage therapist himself, but was afraid to work with this injury...Lucy laid quietly in the candlelit room, and I gently held her injured shoulder in my hands. Within about two minutes, I felt Lucy's breath begin to deepen...I began to use a Brazilian energy clearing technique that I had learned from my Esalen teacher, Maria Lucia Sauer: without touching the body, I felt for hot spots—areas containing excess energy—on the shoulder, grabbed them in my hand, and flung them away. I continued to do this for a couple of minutes, until the area no longer felt hot. By this time Lucy had fallen into a deep sleep.

I then began to do Esalen® Massage, working gently all over the back of Lucy's body, avoiding any pressure in the area of her injured muscle. I used shiatsu pressure on the right arm, to help open the arm energetically to facilitate more clearing in the shoulder. After 20 or 30 minutes, while I was still working on her back, Lucy woke up. She said, ["]I was sleeping! I can't believe I fell asleep, I haven't been able to sleep all week.["] She then checked in with her shoulder, and realized that the pain was gone. She felt so relieved to be pain free that she started to cry.

Because Lucy's shoulder was still injured, the inflammation and pain returned within a couple of days. Lucy continued coming to see me once every two or three days for a 30-minute tune-up to keep the inflammation level low, for a couple of weeks until she had surgery.

The above quote is one of several posted on Peacehope Healing Arts' website. As a licensed massage therapist in practice since 2004, I've had the opportunity to perform massages on a wide variety of clients. After their massage, most clients remark that they feel better, typically commenting that their bodies feel more relaxed (in some cases less anxious), looser, more limber, lighter—especially their necks, shoulders, arms and legs—and they became more positive in their thinking. Numerous clients also mention that simple "touch" made them feel more "grounded," with some going so far as to say, "You have miracle hands."

I was particularly impressed by an experience with a client who had just lost her mother-in-law who had been a major support figure in her life. After a few minutes of massage, she began to cry and told me how much she appreciated my "safe" and "healing" touch. My massage seemed to "free" her—to literally allow her to "get in touch" with—her loss, pain and sadness, in the end providing her with substantial relief. In short, massage helped her to realize her feelings and emotions, despite the depth of her loss. I eventually began to wonder whether it was the massage or her talking that provided the basis for her relief. It was, however, the laying on of hands that to my recollection, brought up her feelings and provided her with the opportunity to release pent up muscular energy and allow her energy to flow. The talking that occurred afterwards seemed more mental self-reflection and closure than traditional psychotherapy. All in all, it was then that I began regularly questioning if whether the laying on of hands might be the primary effect and the talking an after-effect, a "symptom" if you will, of energy flow reestablishment. Shades of Wilhelm Reich! Was this an epiphany or a moment of craziness?

This was reinforced when I read a 1 February 2012, article in *Science Translational Medicine* by Justin D. Crane et al, entitled, "Massage Therapy Attenuates Inflammatory Signaling After Exercise-Induced Muscle Damage," reporting measurable decreases in inflammatory compounds and increased healing in massaged muscles that had experienced hard exercise. Maybe my idea wasn't so crazy after all!

Approaching a Definition of Somatic Therapy

If one were to do an internet search on "somatic therapy," a surprising number of different definitions would appear. Some are similar in nature to Mosby's definition on page 616 of "therapeutic change:" "modification of physical form or function that can affect a client's physical, mental, and/or spiritual state." There are on the other hand, few definitions that agree. Most of these errant definitions are loose and broad-based attempts at defining somatic or body-based *psychotherapy*. For example, the United States Association for Body Psychotherapy defines body psychotherapy as "an expansive field that draws from many eras and traditions—the ancient traditions of intuitive and natural healing, the somatic psychotherapies developed by Wilhelm Reich and others, the American Dance Therapy tradition, the psychoanalytic field, and the more modern traditions of Humanistic, Existential, and Phenomenological psychology." But is somatic *[psycho]therapy* the same as *somatic* therapy?

According to the *American Heritage Medical Dictionary*, somatic refers to "soma" which is defined as: (1) the entire body of an organism, exclusive of germ cells, (2) the axial part of a body, including the head, neck, trunk, and tail, (3) the body of a person as contrasted with the mind or psyche, and/or (4) cell body. There are three important points here. First, soma or somatic involves all the body cells *except the germ cells*. This definition specifically excludes gene therapy, which is often called "somatic gene therapy." Second, soma or somatic *doesn't focus necessarily on thoughts or behaviors* like psychology does. It doesn't exclude psychology, but psychology isn't its main focus. Third, soma or somatic, while it can also refer to an individual body cell, commonly *refers to an organism's entire body*. This dual, combined cellular and holistic focus is important in understanding what somatic therapy actually is.

In Dan Hanlon Johnson's *Bone, Breath, & Gesture - Practices of Embodiment*, Thomas Hanna on page 345 of a chapter entitled "What Is Somatics" expanded on this definition. Hanna, a philosopher and practitioner of the Feldenkrais Method who later established his own approach said, "the distinctiveness of the human soma, is, then, that it is both self-sensing and self-moving and that these interlocked functions are at the core of somatic self-organization and adaptation." Soma and somatics, in Hanna's mind, were closely related to body sensing (e.g. Jacobson's and Levine's "felt sense") and movement. Furthermore, alterations in the soma reflected physiological and anatomical alterations in cellular through organism-level structures.

Integrative social psychotherapist Carole Shepherd, LCSW-R, LMT, RYT, who claims to do "somatic therapy," on her 2011 website, "Integrative Psychotherapy for Balanced Living," categorizes "somatic therapy" as a "complimentary [sic] therapy" alongside thoughtful meditation and yoga therapy. If this is so, then what is a complementary therapy?

On its website, the National Center for Complementary and Alternative Medicine (NCCAM) defines complementary and alternative medicine (CAM) as a broad and constantly changing collection of somatic-based therapies. However, NCCAM also includes in this definition diverse medical and health care systems, practices and products. These therapies, systems, practices and products are not generally considered part of conventional medicine. NCCAM further designates conventional (Western or allopathic) medicine as a system of diagnosis and treatment practiced by holders of MD and DO (doctor of osteopathy) degrees in conjunction with allied health professionals, such as physical therapists, psychologists and registered nurses. CAM therapies include natural products, mind-body medicine, and manipulative and body-based practices. Although these categories are not always formally defined, they are presented to facilitate discussions of CAM practices. In the end, many CAM practices fit into more than one category.

Of the different categories of CAM therapies, mind-body practices focus specifically on interactions between the body, brain, mind, and behavior. CAM therapies listed included meditation, acupuncture, mind-body practices, including deep-breathing exercises, guided imagery, hypnotherapy, progressive relaxation, qi gong, Reiki, Tai chi, Yoga, manipulative and body-based practices, massage therapy, Feldenkrais Method, Alexander Technique and Rolfing. Unfortunately, which, if any, are primary somatic therapies is not clearly indicated. Worse, few of these CAM therapies fit Hanna's characterization of a self-sensing and self-moving process where alterations in the soma would be reflected in physiological and anatomical alterations in bodily structure, then thinking. The question then reduces down to which, if any, of these CAM therapies is intrinsically somatic, or to ask this more precisely, what is necessary to call a therapy "somatic?"

While the attempt to address the "somatic" in *somatic* therapy is of primary importance, it is secondarily, and perhaps even equally important to understand what is meant by the word "therapy."

The *American Heritage Medical Dictionary* defines therapy as "1, The treatment of illness or disability. 2, Psychotherapy. 3, A healing power or quality." This broad, functional definition, similar to the common definitions of "somatic therapy," suggests that all therapies, irrespective of their nature, involve somatic, medical and psychological components. On the other hand, according to the 2011 edition of Biblios, an online resource for the translation from ancient Greek to modern English, the root Greek word θεραπεία, literally *therapeia*, means care or attention, especially medical attention (hence, the similar term, treatment) focused on the reversal of a physical condition, illness or disease. That is, in terms of root definition, therapy, like somatic, refers specifically to the physical body.

A Brief History of Somatic Therapy Redefined

Many different practices claim to be somatic therapies: acupressure, Alexander Technique, anma, body work, bone setting, Bowen Technique, Cranio-sacral Therapy, Dorn Method, Healing Touch, joint manipulation, joint mobilization, massage therapy, myofascial release, Naprapathy, osteopathic manipulation, physical therapy, Rolfing, Seitai, Shiatsu, Sotai, spinal manipulation, spinal mobilization, traction and Tui na.

Probably the oldest of these is massage therapy. According to health writer Paul Hata's 2008 online article, "Massage Therapy - History and Development," posted on Articlesbase.com, massage therapy began to be recognized as a distinct treatment around 3000 BCE in Egypt, India and China. The Chinese at this time collated and codified the various massage techniques of ancient times in the *Cong-Fu of the Tao-Tse*, the oldest known book about massage.

About 1000 BCE, Chinese monks brought massage to Japan, which the Japanese called anma and developed into shiatsu, an energy-building technique to prevent illness, and into acupressure, a technique to bring recipients back into physical and emotional balance, nowadays called homeostasis.

In 500 BCE, the Greek physician, Hippocrates, known today as the "Father of Medicine," used "friction" to heal physical injuries, promoting a combination of massage, proper diet, exercise, rest, fresh air and music to restore bodies to health. The Roman physician, Galen, recommended massage to treat a wide variety of physical ailments. Both the Greeks and Romans used massage to relieve pain in athletes.

It wasn't until the 1700s and the Great Reformation that European scientists rediscovered massage, and even then, it was largely dismissed. Hata reports that in the early 1800s, the Swedish physician Per Henrik Ling developed the Swedish Gymnastic Movement System. This system incorporated "medical" gymnastics and physiology. Techniques included stroking, pressing and squeezing to manually treat physical issues. This form of massage later took the name Swedish massage.

Dr. Sigmund Freud, the father of psychoanalysis and chief proponent of talk therapy, is said to have experimented with massage therapy to treat hysteria.

In *Groundworks - Narrative of Embodiment*, edited by Don Hanlon Johnson, published in 1997, various key second generation somatic therapists summarize how the 1900s saw the rise of numerous different massage therapy methods, for example, the Japanese method, Jin Shin Jyutsu, developed by Jiro Murai to increase circulation, followed quickly by F. M. Alexander's Alexander Technique, Moshe Feldenkrais's Feldenkrais Method, Richard Heckler's Lomi Work, and Dr. Ida Rolf's Deep Tissue Massage, later called Rolfing.

Darcy Elman on page 101 of her chapter, "F. M. Alexander" in Johnson's *Groundworks*, relates that the Alexander Technique was a method of "reeducating people in how they use themselves both in the ordinary activities of daily life (walking, sitting, standing, speaking) and their special activities (singing, rowing, keyboarding), with the goal of creating more ease and freedom from strain." The Feldenkrais Method used directed touch and physical movement to improve human development and function; other methods were also developed, most attempting a more inclusive and comprehensive approach, including such techniques as meditation, group processes, body work, psychotherapy and martial arts.

John P. Conger, in his 1994 book, *The Body in Recovery: Somatic Psychotherapy and the Self*, along with "A Life Chronology," relating the life of Fritz Perls posted on Gestalt.org, state that from 1920 through 1957, Dr. Wilhelm Reich, a student of Freud and psychoanalyst of Fritz Perls of Gestalt Therapy fame, pioneered a form of "psychological body therapy" that was to later be known as somatic therapy. Reich challenged Freud on the validity of "talk therapy" as a primary therapy, holding instead that neuroses were physically located in the tissues of the body where they were expressed as physical rigidity. He believed that only a significant somatic event had the power to entirely release this rigidity which Reich called "body armor." According to the Wilhelm Reich Museum's online biography of Wilhelm Reich, Reich researched Chinese Qi (Ki), calling it orgone energy, and attempted to physically define what it was, and to locate where and how it traveled within the human body.

On page 184 of Janine Chasseguet-Smirgel and Bela Grunberger's *Freud or Reich? Psychoanalysis and Illusion*, translated by Claire Pajaczkowska and published in 1986, the authors state that according to Reich, the "natural" way to reestablish orgone energy flow was through sexual orgasm, as "inhibited sexual energy turns into destructive energy." Reich is said to have frequently alluded to the concept that when one fixes his or her body, (e.g. with massage or some other body therapy), the mind is secondarily fixed as well. This is the basic tenant of modern somatic therapy.

The Wilhelm Reich Museum's website states that Reich closely observed his clients' "natural" movements and reactions to somatic stimuli, and in the process, formulated a series of proscribed physical interventions.

Carl Jung is said to claim, in the 1970 edition of *The Structure and Dynamics of the Psyche Collected Works of C. G. Jung, Volume 8*, that he encouraged his patients to dance out thoughts that proved difficult to put into words. Jung felt that body movements could trigger physically embedded psychological problems, that the tissues were the physical repository of these psychological problems, and that proscribed movements could "release" these problems. This resulted in a wave of interest in dance, and dance movement therapy began to sweep the world.

According to the American Dance Therapy Association (ADTA), modern dancer Maria Chace (aka Marian Chace) established Dance Movement Therapy ostensibly as a somatic therapy, but later allowed it to develop into a humanistic counseling therapy. Sharon Chaiklin, in a 2009 article entitled "Marian Chace: Dancer & Pioneer Dance Therapist," posted on the ADTA website, stated that Chace used individual modern dance (technically not a somatic therapy based on touch), but also couple-contact ballroom dancing (a definite form of somatic therapy) for helping patients recover from both physical and psychological illnesses, injuries and diseases.

Another offspring of Reich's work includes Therapeutic Touch, one Japanese version of which is called Reiki. In either case, the client is physically touched, something Reich experimented with. Yet another is Non-Contact Therapeutic Touch which includes at the extreme, Distance Healing. Developed in the 1970s by Dora Kunz, a theosophy promoter, and Dolores

Krieger, a nursing educator at New York University, Distance Healing was said to be an energy therapy that promoted healing and reduced pain and anxiety. As with Reiki therapy, hands—either the client's in self-therapy, or a practitioner's—are placed on or near the target area in order to manipulate the patient's energy field. The Reiki process is well-described by the International Center for Reiki Training on its website at Reiki.org.

In the past, therapeutic efficacy claims regarding various somatic therapies were mostly based on anecdotal reports. However, increasing emphasis is being placed on the ability to scientifically demonstrate efficacy. For example, in a 1998 study reported in the prestigious *Journal of the American Medical Association* by Linda Rosa RN, Emily Rosa, Larry Sarner and Stephen Barrett MD entitled, "A Close Look at Therapeutic Touch," twenty-one experienced Therapeutic Touch practitioners were unable to detect the presence or absence of a hand placed a few inches above theirs with their vision obstructed. This suggests, at least, that detection of energy fields "from a distance" may not be possible, thus limiting somatic therapy to skin-to-skin touch.

In summary, somatic therapy, at its core, includes human-to-human, skin-to-skin contact and the direct physical results of that contact. Somatic therapy is neither a form of psychology (in terms of the study of behavior or thinking), nor a cognitive-based psychotherapy. While psychological applications and cognitive therapies may include elements or even the whole of somatic therapy, they are not somatic therapy *per se*. This reorientation is absolutely necessary for somatic therapy to change from a loose group of "pop" psychological practices and approaches to a rich, robust and researchable science of its own.

Somatic therapy is the treatment of illness, injury or disease in humans (and technically other animals, and one could even imagine plants) through direct touch contact. Somatic therapy, at its pinnacle, would likewise include the prevention of illness, injury or disease through the direct laying on of hands.

In short, somatic therapy includes those practices involving self and person-to-person contact that are intended to prevent, heal or help a person to recover from illness, injury or disease.

My Thoughts and Observations about the Science of Somatic Therapy

This reoriented definition of somatic therapy includes massage, acupressure (but not necessarily acupuncture) and contact Dance Movement Therapy. These therapies involve touching, pushing, pulling, stroking, rubbing, tapping and patting. Swedish massage, for example, uses five strokes, including *effleurage* (sliding or gliding), *petrissage* (kneading), *tapotement* (tapping), along with frictional (cross fiber) and vibratory shaking.

Whether or not somatic therapies, as defined above, have an effect on the body is no longer in question. Terry M. Levy and Michael Orlans, in their groundbreaking 1988 medical text entitled, *Attachment, Trauma, and Healing*, claimed that mammals are born with an innate need to be affectionately touched and stroked. Affectionate touch and stroking is correlated with better brain development, increased weight gain, greater activity and resilience under stress. To this, Shiela Koty Globus in her 2002 article, "Touch Me I'm Yours: The Benefits of Infant Massage" published in *Special Delivery* added that such touching and stroking stimulates the nerves, increases blood flow and strengthens the immune system.

For example, according to a NCCAM report summarizing an article entitled, "A preliminary study of the effects of a single session of Swedish massage on hypothalamic-pituitary-adrenal and immune function in normal individuals," published in *The Journal of Alternative and Complementary Medicine* in 2010, researchers from Cedars-Sinai Medical Center and the David Geffen School of Medicine at the University of California Los Angeles randomly assigned 53 healthy adults to receive one session of either Swedish massage or light touch. A licensed massage therapist delivered the somatic therapy for 45 minutes. Blood samples taken before and after the sessions showed that participants who received Swedish massage had a significant decrease in the hormone arginine-vasopressin (which plays a role in regulating blood pressure and water retention) compared with those who were treated with light touch. Significant decreases in cytokines (interleukin 4 and interleukin 10), but not others (interleukin 1 beta, interleukin 2, interleukin 5, and tumor necrosis factor alpha), were found in the massage group compared to the light touch group. These preliminary data led the researchers to conclude that a single session of Swedish massage can produce measurable biological effects, affecting both hormone (emotional) and immune systems as well.

Acupressure is an ancient healing art where the practitioner uses his or her fingers to press on key points on an imaginary meridian line projected in the practitioner's mind onto the surface of the skin. In a 25 March 2006 *British Medical Journal* article entitled, "Treatment of low back pain by acupressure and physical therapy: randomized controlled trial," by Lisa Li-Chen Hsieh *et al*, acupressure conferred an 89% reduction in disability compared with physical therapy, after adjusting for pretreatment disability. This improvement lasted for six months. Similar benefits were reported for "leg pain."

More recently, *MedPage Today* Senior Staff Writer Crystal Phend, in a 13 February 2011 online article entitled, "ASA: Senses Stoke Stroke Recovery," reported a study by University of California Irvine PhD candidate Melissa F. Davis showing that rat-whisker stimulation started within 10 minutes of a stroke protected brain function by increasing blood flow through collateral vessels. Stimulating more whiskers led to faster recovery, Davis and her team claimed. Touching areas like the fingers and lips could be inferred to have a similar effect on the human brain.

Reexamined and redefined in the above way, *somatic* therapy (as distinguished from somatic *therapy*) is quite amenable to scientific research, allowing an increasingly clearer understanding of its effects and benefits.

In conclusion, the search for somatic therapy is a difficult and elusive one. There are many different definitions of somatic therapy supported by different interest groups, the principal group being counseling psychologists attempting to fold the results of somatic therapies into the psychological and cognitive realms.

This has resulted, in the author's opinion, in the loss of a clear definition of somatic therapy. Instead, the author offers a richer, more robust, focused and researchable definition that will clarify the preventive and healing effects of somatic therapies involving skin-to-skin touch, whether superficial or deep, either alone or in association with muscle, lymphatic or bone manipulation, or other sensory therapies involving visual (sight), auditory (sound), olfactory (smell), and/or gustatory (taste) senses. For example, dance therapy, art therapy, music therapy, aromatherapy, and taste therapy, when they occur without skin-to-skin touch, would not be considered somatic therapies. This new definition also expands the concept of somatic therapy to include therapies involving self and/or person-to-person "skin-to-skin" touch. Reich early on realized the importance of what some would call "sexual contact" and experimented with this form of somatic therapy against prevailing social mores. How then, does one include this modality while protecting the client from sexual trauma and abuse? According to Dr. Daniel S. Janik, in his 2005 book entitled, *Unlock the Genius Within: Neurobiological Trauma, Teaching and Transformative Learning*, non-abusive touch is "wanted" touch. Janik argues that self or interpersonal skin-to-skin "wanted" touch does not fall within the definition of trauma or abuse. While this forward approach, like Reich's early work, pushes prevailing social and professional ethical limits, it provides for the investigation, research, development and practice of a broader somatic therapy. This expanded definition is not without recognition of such areas of somatic therapy as the ritual practice of tantric yoga and Esalen's explorations in tantric massage.

Setsuko Tsuchiya

Chapter 15
Changing Somatic Therapy

I've always been interested in the human body: how it works, why it fails and what can help it to heal and prevent it from failing. I've learned through my studies at Hawaii College of Health Sciences from 2003 to 2004, where I worked with both a licensed medical doctor, Dr. Daniel S. Janik, and a licensed doctor of osteopathy, Dr. Randall H. James, that there is a difference between disease and illness. Disease is an abnormal condition affecting an organism. Illness is about feelings—like pain, fatigue, weakness, discomfort, distress, confusion, or dysfunction—that may or may not accompany disease, and is the way most people judge the effectiveness of treatment. Illness typically, but not always, accompanies disease as in the case of a highly aggressive and lethal "silent" cancer. A treatment or therapy can seemingly not work when in fact, it is, and conversely it may seem to work when in fact, it isn't. Somatic therapists, like massage therapists, should always be careful to separate disease from illness, for example by asking a client if he or she has seen a licensed physician for any underlying conditions and whether the doctor has ordered, or at least allows, somatic therapy. Massage, for example, can help people recover faster, better and easier from illnesses. Diseases, on the other hand, commonly require medication or surgery in order for the person to be healed. In summary, I became interested in the human body, and both my dancing and my medical massage practice from 2004 to present has helped me better understand the nature of *somatic* therapy—what I would call "somatic therapy" in general—and what I do in a broader sense.

I began taking psychology courses to help me understand where exactly mind and body meet. How do illnesses in the mind affect diseases in the body? Similarly, how do diseases affect illnesses? My classes in General Psychology, as well as Psychological Foundations of Eurythmic Therapies, Basic Movement in DMT, Progressive Muscle Relaxation, and History and Systems of Psychology all helped me to get a better grasp of the complex relationship between the body and mind.

Studying psychology, I was surprised to learn about the importance of neurobiology. This seems to me to be at the heart of all illness and somatic therapy. I learned that the ancient Greeks recognized the physical and as a result, mental healing qualities of body movement (though they would have regarded it dance eurythmia) and decided to become a Dance Movement Therapist. In my Basic Movement in DMT class, I came to realize that DMT as a whole is not yet well understood. It has yet to recognize any basic healing movements (a surprise), and DMT treatments are not yet widely neurobiologically-based (a disappointment). I learned about the split between clinical and counseling psychology, and that counseling psychology included somatic therapy which included many "body-based" psychotherapies including DMT. I wasn't completely sure how these different therapies related to massage therapy, DMT, actual somatic therapy or psychological counseling.

I slowly came to realize that complementary and alternative medical (CAM) therapies, when used in conjunction with counseling psychology, are loosely called somatic therapy—though perhaps better, specialized counseling—and when used in association with human touch and bodywork could truthfully be called somatic therapy. So, I become more interested in somatic therapy as a career.

After searching, I came to find that there are currently no somatic therapy training programs in Hawaii. Somewhat saddened, but not exactly surprised by the lack of a local program, I began to search for other places where I could study and learn somatic therapy by attendance or even distance education. The closest I came, however, was Naropa University's master's degree in somatic therapy.

When I began undergraduate studies, I acquired some new abilities outside of my knowledge and experience while exploring dance and massage therapy in more detail. I learned, for example, American-style critical thinking. This is especially challenging for someone who was brought up in Japan and had been exposed mainly to Japanese approaches to thinking and analysis. However, I perceived that I would need this ability to complete a master's degree in somatic therapy. Having completed my undergraduate studies, I felt like I was beginning to understand this uniquely American way of investigating and evaluating what I read and heard.

I learned through my undergraduate and graduate research that I don't actually need another license in Hawaii to practice somatic therapy—my massage license is enough. This further fueled my desire for more education in somatic therapy. I'm still exploring how I would use this knowledge in my current dance and massage practices. For example, should I expand the scope of my massage therapy practice or actually change to being a "somatic therapist" using massage, DMT, Rolfing, Ki, and other forms of somatic therapy combined with muscle relaxation, deep breathing and yoga?

I also realized I know a lot more than I thought about the muscles of the body, body movement and neurobiology. This happened again and again during meetings of the Neurobiological Learning Society. Even my earliest attempts to separate the effects of the laying on of hands from "talk therapy" proved insightful and challenging, not only to myself, but everyone I talked with. These experiences helped me to attain a new level of confidence in my abilities and my search to become an outstanding somatic therapist.

While my core values, such as my desire to help people, haven't changed, my understanding of and appreciation for the power of somatic therapy have. For example, I have come to value prevention over treatment. I would like to help prevent illnesses (and quite possibly diseases) before they happen. I'm not sure yet how to do this, but I am certain this is important. Finally, in the end, I want to take what I learn about somatic therapy and share it with practitioners and people in my native country, Japan.

In a strange about-face, my search for somatic therapy has left me less interested in DMT than I was before. Still, I would like to be part of DMT's continued development. For example, I would like to reintroduce couples social dance into DMT as a preventive somatic therapy, but I want it to include basic movements that include characteristics of somatic therapy that are neurobiologically relevant.

I have also come to respect Rolfers and the emphasis they place on oral therapy, breathing and posture, though I'm interested not just in static posture, but moving posture—what I've come to believe is the "real" basis for the somatic part of DMT and somatic therapy, as long as it involves self or person-to-person, skin-to-skin contact.

At the same time, I don't want to limit my professional knowledge and development simply to massage or DMT. I want to expand my current practice to include more somatic-based approaches such as progressive relaxation, neuromuscular touch and somatic movement using the fundamentals of somatic therapy and the new neurobiological/medical (CAM) model described earlier. This approach should open new doors in somatic therapy, for instance, somatic stimulation might help humans more completely heal from a stroke or maybe even help prevent a stroke altogether.

In short, I feel more and more confident about somatic therapy as a professional pursuit and a future career as a somatic therapist.

Before I undertook this journey—my search for somatic therapy—I had a feeling that I might want to change my career from that of a registered medical massage therapist to that of a dance movement therapist. Now, I've begun to change my mind again. As part of my journey, I researched the Dictionary of Occupational Titles (DOT), *Occupational Outlook Handbook* (DOH), Monster Board, Monstertrak and joined both the American Dance Therapy Association (ADTA) and Japan Dance Therapy Association (JADTA). When I looked for "dance movement therapist" in the DOT and DOH, I was surprised to not find it listed. Then I looked for "massage therapist" and was even more surprised to not find it either. I did, however, locate physical therapy and recreational therapy, both of which include somatic elements as well as "talk" therapy. These aren't what I'm interested in, but the implication seemed clear to me: My future remains clearly with the somatic part of somatic therapy!

Towards the end of my search, I reinterviewed three people: Dr. Daniel S. Janik MD PhD, Dr. Lewis Mehl-Madrona MD PhD, and Ms. Barbara Mainguy MA, all experts in different areas of somatic therapy. As a consequence, and in association with my own search, I discovered that massage therapy and dance movement therapy represent only two of many possible forms of somatic therapy. I am now interested in pursuing somatic therapy, stressing the somatic part, as a career rather than massage or some form of dance movement therapy. Furthermore, when I corresponded with members of ADTA and JADTA, I learned that somatic therapy continues to move in the direction of that which is somatic, especially neurobiological, while Dance Movement Therapy is increasingly becoming a therapeutic art form, incorporating more and more talk therapy into its process.

English is still a problem for me, so I am even more interested in using somatic therapy because it is a more "hands-on" rather than psychological counseling approach requiring an extensive and subtle command of a particular culture and its language. I would like to be one of the pioneers who uncover the basic, fundamental somatic elements of somatic therapy, elements like deep breathing, self and/or person-to-person touch, natural movement, correct posture, progressive relaxation and couples movement and interaction.

I look forward to expanding my current practice, working towards further redefining somatic therapy, and bringing this idea to the forefront in the USA, Japan and the rest of the world. I think that the Japanese will be particularly interested in somatic therapy, as Eastern medicine, Yoga, Reiki, Ki and Tai-chi are already familiar to the Japanese. Somatic therapy, in the sense that I have redefined it, seems to me, a next logical step.

My long-range career goal at recent is to become a pioneer practitioner-consultant of somatic therapy for Pacific Rim countries, including my home country of Japan. I am already considering joining and helping further develop national and international somatic therapy associations like the International Somatic Movement Education and Therapy Association.

As the world continues to advance technologically, especially in the workplace, people will undoubtedly experience increasing stress, so knowledge and wisdom regarding the application of preventive somatic therapy will likely become increasingly important. CAM therapies are just beginning to be appreciated; Western and Eastern medicine, I think, will continue to slowly come together and result in a whole new understanding of illness and disease based around stress, stress amelioration and stress prevention.

In getting to this place in my career, I tried to incorporate careful research, strategic planning, critical thinking and intuitive guidance. At the moment, I feel good about both the process and direction of my pathway and look forward to continuing my journey in search of somatic therapy.

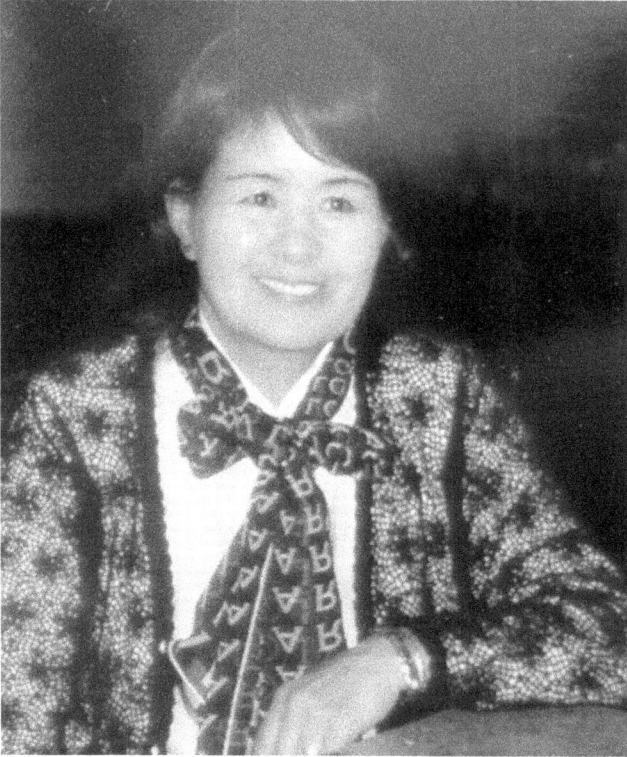

About the Author

Originally from Japan, Setsuko Tsuchiya immigrated to the USA, earned a BA in Liberal Arts in Dance from Thomas Edison University, while studying medical massage therapy at Hawaii College of Health Sciences. A DanceSport athlete and competitive dancer, after becoming a licensed medical massage therapist, she began wondering if there might be such a thing as a fundamental somatic (body) basis for the burgeoning number of body-based therapies, one that is independent of language and applicable to all cultures in this increasingly globalized world. She is an honored fellow of the American Association of Integrative Medicine.

Index

A

77-78, 85, 113-115, 120, 140, 142-143, 148-149, 151-152, 155, 171, 182, 195
cred(it/ited/ential), 89, 121, 135, 143
Crisp, 13-15, 19-21, 36, 45, 127, 143
criteri(a/on), 33, 52
criti(cal/cize/cism/cized), 17, 131-132, 156, 207, 212
Crozier, 15
Cruz, 149
cry, 188
CSD, 136-137
Cuba(n), 14, 16, 18, 53, 62-63, 67, 74, 79
Cugat, 16
cultur(e/es/al), 36-37, 84, 86, 110, 122-124, 127-128, 136, 139, 211, 213
cur(e/ative), 96, 120,
Curcurruto, 181
cycl(e/es/ic/cal), 97, 183
cytokines, 200

D

Dalcroze, 142, 152
Danc(es/ed/ing/able/er/ers incl *danse* and DanceSport), 1-71, 73-85, 87-91, 93-97, 108-111, 113-117, 119-123, 125, 127-128, 131-137, 139-145, 148-161, 163-164, 166-167, 180, 185, 190, 197, 199, 202, 206-211, 213
Dan(tian/tien), 166
Davis, 201
death(s), 94, 97, 140
debilitating, 181
defens(e/es/ive) 16, 99, 103, 171, 174
defin(es/ed/ition/itions/itive), 1-2, 20-21, 25, 27-28, 31, 33-35, 43, 46, 52-54, 57, 68, 77, 83, 90, 140, 146, 149, 151, 155-159, 161, 167, 172, 177, 189-193, 196, 199, 201-203

E

F

G

H

J

K

L

M

133, 148, 155-156, 165-166, 169, 171, 176, 185, 187-189, 192-196, 199-200, 203, 205-211, 213

McAllister, 6

McCormack, 82

McWilliams, 164-165

medic(al/ally,ine/ations), 1-2, 47, 89, 95, 99-100, 102, 106-107, 117, 126, 136, 140, 145-146, 148, 150, 156, 166, 189-194, 198-201, 205-207, 209-213

meditat(ion/tive), 126, 182, 191-192, 195

Mehl(-Madrona), 210

melody, 36, 54

menstruation, 174

mental(ly incl health), 85-86, 90, 96, 100, 102, 104-106, 112-115, 117, 119-121, 123-128, 134-135, 146-147, 156, 171-172, 175, 179, 179, 182, 189-190, 206

merengue, 23-24

meridian(s), 90, 106, 166-167, 201

Merriam(-Webster), 35

Mezger, 39

microspasms, 90

Min, 83

mind, 54, 95-97, 107-108, 112, 115-116, 127-128, 136, 139, 141, 153, 156, 165-166, 173, 175, 179, 190-192, 196, 201, 206, 210

Miranda, 19

modern (incl British/International ballroom dance), 7, 22, 34-35, 37-39, 43-45, 55, 79, 91, 93-95, 115-116, 120-121, 127, 137, 140, 142-145, 148-153, 158, 190, 193, 196-197

Moore, 22, 58-61, 74

moral(ly), 96, 126, 141

Morita(Therapy), 126

Morsbach, 128

Mosby, 89, 190

motion(s see also move), 15-17, 19, 29, 33, 38, 62-63, 65, 67, 78-79, 83, 89, 169

N

Q

R

T

U

V

valse(see also waltz), 12
[arginine-]vasopressin, 200
vibrat(e/ion/ions/ory), 90, 93-94, 199
victim(s), 101, 184

W

Waibert, 80
waltz(en/es), 4, 7, 9-10, 12-13, 15-16, 22-26, 28, 55-56, 60-61, 66, 71, 114, 120
war, 4, 6-7, 10, 16, 20, 49, 141, 151
WD(C/&DSC), 20, 29, 77
Webber, 164
[Mirriam-]Webster, 34-35
Weiss, 77
West(ern/erners), 4, 15, 17, 36, 42, 45, 90, 106, 111, 119-120, 123, 125-129, 140-141, 156, 166, 192, 212
whisker(s), 201
White, 11
Whitehouse, 111-112, 114, 116, 148, 150-151
Wigman, 149, 152
Wooden, 83

Y

Yacco, 144
YMCA, 4, 74
yoga, 107, 191-192, 203, 208, 211

If you enjoyed *In Search of Somatic Therapy,* consider these other fine books from Savant Books and Publications:

Essay, Essay, Essay by Yasuo Kobachi

Aloha from Coffee Island by Walter Miyanari

Footprints, Smiles and Little White Lies by Daniel S. Janik

The Illustrated Middle Earth by Daniel S. Janik

Last and Final Harvest by Daniel S. Janik

A Whale's Tale by Daniel S. Janik

Tropic of California by R. Page Kaufman

Tropic of California (the companion music CD) by R. Page Kaufman

The Village Curtain by Tony Tame

Dare to Love in Oz by William Maltese

The Interzone by Tatsuyuki Kobayashi

Today I Am a Man by Larry Rodness

The Bahrain Conspiracy by Bentley Gates

Called Home by Gloria Schumann

Kanaka Blues by Mike Farris

First Breath edited by Z. M. Oliver

Poor Rich by Jean Blasiar

The Jumper Chronicles by W. C. Peever

William Maltese's Flicker by William Maltese

My Unborn Child by Orest Stocco

Last Song of the Whales by Four Arrows

Perilous Panacea by Ronald Klueh

Falling but Fulfilled by Zachary M. Oliver

Mythical Voyage by Robin Ymer

Hello, Norma Jean by Sue Dolleris

Richer by Jean Blasiar

Manifest Intent by Mike Farris

Charlie No Face by David B. Seaburn

Number One Bestseller by Brian Morley

My Two Wives and Three Husbands by S. Stanley Gordon

In Dire Straits by Jim Currie

Wretched Land by Mila Komarnisky

Chan Kim by Ilan Herman

Who's Killing All the Lawyers? by A. G. Hayes

Ammon's Horn by G. Amati

Wavelengths edited by Zachary M. Oliver

Almost Paradise by Laurie Hanan

Communion by Jean Blasiar and Jonathan Marcantoni

The Oil Man by Leon Puissegur

Random Views of Asia from the Mid-Pacific by William E. Sharp

The Isla Vista Crucible by Reilly Ridgell

Blood Money by Scott Mastro

In the Himalayan Nights by Anoop Chandola

On My Behalf by Helen Doan

Traveler's Rest by Jonathan Marcantoni

In Search of Somatic Therapy

www.ingramcontent.com/pod-product-compliance
Lightning Source LLC
Chambersburg PA
CBHW062210270326
41930CB00009B/1699